FINDING FREEDOM

ESCAPING FROM THE PRISON OF CHRONIC FATIGUE SYNDROME

RAELAN AGLE

Finding Freedom:

Escaping from the Prison of

Chronic Fatigue Syndrome

EDITION NOTICE

First paperback edition December 2019
Editing by Dr. D. Olson Pook
Cover design by Miladinka Milic

ISBN: 9781707010196

Visit www.raelanagle.com

CONTENTS

PREFACE

During my long struggle with chronic fatigue syndrome (CFS), despite reading countless books on topics as varied as herbalism and homeopathy, I never found a single book that had all the information I needed to escape this horrific condition. I didn't find one that *even came close.*

I wanted a book that would tell me what it's actually like to live with such a debilitating illness and show me how to endure the many dark and desperate days that were sure to come. I wanted a book that would connect me to a supportive community of other CFS sufferers so that during the time it took to recover I would not be alone. And most of all I wanted a book that showed me beyond a shadow of a doubt that people can and actually do recover and that laid out the step-by-step instructions describing exactly how those people escaped the prison that is CFS — forever.

It took me many years to completely recover from CFS (or myalgic encephalomyelitis as it's also referred to as), and during that long and difficult time I spent tens of thousands of dollars on my health. In the end, I learned that getting better neither had to take anywhere near that long nor cost me anywhere near that much. In fact, regaining my health boiled down to developing some new habits and following some basic guidelines that, when rigorously followed, allowed me to get back my life and my freedom.

So when I finally did recover from CFS, I knew I had to write that book I'd been looking for. The book that would have saved me years of wading through mountains of information (and misinformation) in a desperate search to find what worked and what did not. The book that would have spared me all those tears of frustration when I had more questions than answers and absolutely no idea if what I was doing was helping or hurting. And most of all, the book that I would have given to every other CFS sufferer I knew in the hopes that they would get their freedom back the way I did after reading it.

As the transformation guru Rachel Hollis explains, when humans go through something hard, they react in one of two ways. They come out the other side either better or worse. It's impossible to walk through hell and leave it the same way you went in. Nobody walks through fire unscathed. You either burn up into ashes or you get forged in the flames and emerge as something new.

In this book, during our time together, I want to be with you as you emerge as something new. To be with you as you move forward, find your own unique path out of this while you see your truths and be honest about what's going on, even if it's only to yourself.

I want you to know that you're strong enough to survive this — even on the days that feels impossible. You are strong enough and it is possible to come through the other side as a better version of yourself. [1]

If you or someone you care about is struggling with CFS, I wrote this book for you. I've filled the pages of this book with everything I could think of that helped me through the longest and most difficult season of my life. I wrote this book so that I could share my story and do my part to shed some light on this mysterious illness. I wrote this book to fulfill the promise I made that if I recovered I would do everything in my power to share how I escaped. I wrote this book in the hopes that when reading it, those suffering from CFS might just feel a little bit less alone.

If you're like me, then you've already read every book you can find on the topic of health and healing. I'm not here to regurgitate any of that. You know it all already. What I will share are the concrete strategies that I developed out of years of trial and error that allowed me to finally recover from CFS. Following these strategies has allowed me not only to survive but to thrive. The things I share are all built around one thing: what helped me get my health and my full life back. I hope the insights I share will save you precious time. I hope my years of struggle will fuel and inspire your speedy recovery. And most of all, I hope my experiences help you on your journey out of the pain you are enduring. I know, because I've been there.

And if in the end, my path is not your path, then at the very least then you will have read about the journey that I went on to find my freedom and perhaps this will spark some insight and help point that spotlight of yours in the direction it needs to be for you to forge your own way out of this as well.

Ultimately, the number one thing that will get you past this is perseverance, that ability to keep manifesting hope when all hope seems lost, that focus and drive to keep working while refusing to accept anything less than the vibrant and joyous life that you deserve.

Maybe you've already tried countless things to get yourself better, and you're feeling a little reluctant to get your hopes up again. Perhaps too many failures and too much suffering have made you more than a little skeptical that healing from CFS is even possible. I am here to tell you that for me, recovery *was* possible. I am living, breathing proof that people absolutely can and do get their health back. Not some of it. Not three-quarters of it. *All* of it.

And I want from the depths of my soul for you to achieve this too. I want to be there for you — *with you* — as you turn your struggles into strengths and free yourself from the chains of CFS.

AUTHOR'S NOTE

Aside from slightly altering the timing of some events for simplicity's sake, I have written everything in this book exactly as I remember it. There are a few people listed in this book by name. Some of those names are real, and some have been changed to a pseudonym to preserve anonymity.

I recommend a few specific products and brands in this book by name. At the time of this writing, I have not received any money from any of these sources for their promotion. I mention them with the hope that they might help you as they have me. As with any advice, do your own research and use your own judgment before deciding if they are right for you.

I also at times use gender pronouns such as he or she, but at all times my words and my story are meant to be inclusive of all people.

I know that chronic fatigue syndrome goes by various names such as Myalgic Encephalomyelitis, ME, and ME/CFS. Due to no reason other than habit, I typically refer to it as CFS.

I'm not a doctor, fitness trainer, or certified health professional of any kind. I'm just a regular person whose life was turned upside down by CFS. When I couldn't find treatment advice that worked from medical professionals, I decided that, rather than give up, I would figure out how to beat this illness on my own.

What I share in this book is based on my own research and experimentation and what worked for me. The details of my recovery are given with the express understanding that before trying anything that I mention, you will first talk with a trusted and certified health professional. Nothing in these pages should be construed as medical advice or treatment.

In addition, you should listen to the one CFS expert who knows so much about what is best for your body — YOU.

INTRODUCTION
LESSONS FROM LIFE

Sure, I could jump straight into what worked for me, but I know I need to share my story first. It would certainly be easier for me to simply get straight to what worked for me for chronic fatigue syndrome recovery, and it would be easier in the short term for you to skip straight to that part and read only that, but on both of our parts that would be a mistake. It would be a mistake because without knowing who I am, what I've been through, and how many times I've failed and *how* I failed before finally succeeding, the end result will have little impact. Without understanding how I got to my answers, those answers will never make sense or be credible to you. You're smart and savvy and you're going to want proof that what I'm talking about actually worked for me. The proof is in the pudding, so to speak, and the pudding is my life leading up to my recovery.

We've all had those moments — quick flashes of insight followed up by . . . absolutely nothing. We read an article or watch a clip on YouTube and think we've found the recipe for success, and then it goes no further. A flowchart of suggestions to consider just isn't going to cut it for you. You need to know the dirt and to taste the blood, sweat, and tears that went into getting the result before you can know the truth of what I'm saying.

So instead of diving straight into my own recipe for health and happiness, this book starts with sharing my experiences with pain, fear, sadness, and finally triumph so that I can empower, inspire, motivate, and challenge you to create a success story of your own. I know that the more authentic I am about my struggles with CFS, the better this book will be.

The second reason I share theses stories is because I want them to have meant something. All the struggle, all the suffering, I want it to have been more than random misfortune and a crappy hand in life. These stories, these seasons, they moulded me into someone resilient and magnificent. And I want you to know that your story can and will do the same for you too.

If you have CFS, by reading what I went through you will know in your heart that you are not alone in your struggles. And if you are reading this and you are fortunate enough to have never faced CFS, my story will put a human face on this devastating illness. It will make CFS real to everyone who doesn't understand it and shed some light on what living with chronic illness actually looks like and feels like.

Plus, I want to have some fun in this process! And I bet you do too. I like to laugh, and I *love* to be silly. Just ask most of my past employers. At one of my jobs, there was a rumor going around that I was a psychology student posing as an employee who was there to study how many ridiculous things I could get people to do in the workplace. When I'm in charge of a meeting I bring toys and play music and make people hop around on one foot just for the heck of it because life really is too short to not have some fun while living it. True of office meetings — and true of books as well.

I'll admit, some parts of my story are a bit heavy. This *is*

CFS, after all, so there is just no way around that. But other parts are also so ridiculous and comical that you can't help but laugh. And that glimpse around the corner from someone who's already been down that path you're on might just help you be better prepared to avoid the potholes and road closures that might be coming your way. So start from the beginning, take this journey with me and learn to spot the false saviors, skip the time wasters, and prepare yourself for the good stuff waiting for you in life.

And congratulations on being motivated to start on your transformation. At whatever stage of illness or health you are at, I promise that you will find pieces of this story that will make you laugh while screaming, *Yes! I feel that!* and make you adamant that the status quo of ill health and subpar happiness is absolutely unacceptable. Get ready because we're about to have some fun, probably shed a few tears, and get through this thing *together*.

I

ENTERING THE PRISON

1

THE CRASH

I remember the exact moment I heard the click of the cell door behind me and realized that nothing would ever be the same again. To this day, I can recreate every sensation and every thought as if they were happening all over again. I can still picture the "old me" before she slipped away and disappeared, only to be replaced by the "new me" trapped in a cage I couldn't escape.

Newly diagnosed and standing in the bedroom of our home, I was gazing at the happy faces of my husband and me captured in a framed photograph sitting atop our reclaimed wood dresser. I had an impractical love for this particular dresser. Its drawers were roughly made and oddly shaped, and I struggled every single time I had to open them. The whole thing spanned almost an entire wall and was impossibly heavy — there was no thought ever of moving it against a different wall. But it was exactly the right shade of brown: a shade that had never explicitly been in style, making it unlikely to ever go out of style. At first glance, the dresser appeared rugged and worn as if it had been constructed from old railway ties, but as I ran my hand over it that morning, I took pleasure in its silky lacquered feeling beneath my fingertips.

At that moment in time I was a person who took a great deal of pleasure from material comforts. We were at the start of a typically cold Canadian winter, and as the gas fireplace gently warmed the house, I looked out the bedroom window as the fluffy white snow floated to the ground. The contrast between the icy exterior taking shape and the warmth suffusing through the interior space of my house struck me. Although I treasured every inch of this house, the fireplace was its crown jewel. Its fire blazed from within a two-story open concept living room with an impossibly high ceiling that allowed the twenty-four-foot-high slate-covered fireplace to run all the way up the wall to the top floor of our home. I could feel its warmth in every room in the house, and cozily standing there in front of that beloved dresser should have been one of the happiest moments of my life.

I had always anticipated what moving into a house like this would feel like — a key smoothly turning as the tumblers clicked into place, the final puzzle piece that completed the scene laid out before me. Having only just moved in a couple months prior, the exhilaration of finally living in a place where *grownups* would live had not yet worn off, and I thought it never would. Gone were the days of cheap rental apartments and postage stamp-sized starter homes. Living in this house signified success and substance; it even made me feel more important while I was at work despite not one person there either knowing or caring where I lived. But as my thirtieth birthday was just around the corner, I felt like I definitely had something to prove — and as far I was concerned, the prestige I felt living in this house was proof that I'd finally *arrived*.

So you can imagine what I thought I should have been feeling that early winter's day as I stared absently at our suntanned faces in the photo adorning the dresser top. But instead of the fairy tale existence I had so long planned for, the harsh reality of what was happening to me began to sink in: as I began to focus on the details of that photograph, the woman — that energetic person smiling back at me in the photo — was gone.

As I transferred my gaze from the photograph and looked at myself in the full-length bedroom mirror, I could literally feel my material successes fade in significance. It's not just that they diminished in importance; I could *feel* them become insubstantial, like ghosts haunting a past life. All that was left to me was my body. I looked intently in the mirror and took stock of my suddenly most prized possession.

The mirror still showed my taut muscles, flat stomach, and flab-less arms. With all this body sculpting, some evidence of my having cheekbones had even emerged from my stubbornly round face, with its deep brown eyes that sparkled out from my frustratingly fine yet glossy chin-length brown locks. Everything stretched out beautifully slim and lean, tight and appealing: from my slender neck and my elegant fingers all the way down to my long and narrow feet. If there is, in fact, such a thing as being *big boned*, then I was definitely the poster girl for being *small boned*. With my tapered ribcage and trim core, people have actually pondered where my organs could possibly fit. My Lululemon yoga pants — an absolute staple of my wardrobe in those days — still fit like a glove while highlighting all the right curves. The pricey black Lycra showed off my legs for days, culminating in a firm and high backside that for most women (after the teen years have passed) is a trophy that must be earned before it can be prominently displayed. Even with the typical feelings of self-doubt, I couldn't deny that I looked strong and powerful and capable of taking on anything.

Here's where I heard it — the cell door of my illness locking behind me — and suddenly I could see through the lies that that mirror told. A sickening realization crept over me: the fit body the mirror was reflecting back at me, the one I had obsessed for hours over maintaining, had become a thing of the past; it was about to join the other ghosts that haunted my house. I saw my future self unfold in front of me: weak muscles, a gross and flabby mid-section, and sad little arms. My dim eyes and recessed cheekbones now invisible amid my bulbous face, with a double chin setting the pace for what was to come down the rest of my drooping body. Everything sagged; nothing was sexy. My yoga pants would still be a staple, but they'd be worn due to their stretchy and accommodating nature, showcasing what I insensitively thought of as *Mom Bum* in place of my fit derrière. Looking in the mirror, I felt weak and powerless and incapable of managing anything at all.

It's more than a little embarrassing to admit that *this* was what I was thinking about when I finally admitted to myself that I wasn't just feeling ill or run down. But looking back, maybe it's not surprising that it took so long for me to concede that something far more serious was happening to my body if this was the cost of that realization. Because there was something even worse than simply losing who I was — it was watching my life start to mirror the contours of someone else's, a life I knew too well, and undergoing a transformation that I would have done anything to prevent.

As I accepted the illness revealing itself to me in the mirror, I slowly inhaled a breath, released it with defeat, and silently said my goodbyes. Not to my health. Somehow I couldn't focus on that; I wasn't there yet. What I am ashamed to admit is that what I said goodbye to was my ability to live a life in service of my *vanity*. Three months before my thirtieth birthday, I could no longer complete even five measly sit-ups on my bedroom floor. My plan to commit to a daily workout of just ten simple squats each morning from my favorite spot in our upstairs loft had failed miserably. From beginner's yoga poses to simple living room workouts designed for aging seniors, I'd failed at completing them all. It had become decisively clear to me that the levels of exertion required to keep my sculpted body were now far more than I could manage. But it took this moment in time for me to accept it.

That was the moment when I finally conceded that my fitness-obsessed life was officially and indefinitely on hold. My days of slaying boot camp and rocking kick-boxing classes were behind me. No more pre-dawn ten-kilometer runs before work. No more grueling personal trainer sessions lifting weights and running the stairs. No more action-packed fitness classes with legions of other obsessed athletes where I exited the exercise room with an exhausted yet satisfied grin on my face. I could no longer deny it. I was ill.

I took a long look at the face in the mirror as my jailer sent the bolt echoing home. At thirty, my life as I knew it was over.

Looking back at my family history I should have known something like this was bound to happen, but I had hoped that the family curse would skip a generation. The first member of my family struck down was my maternal grandmother. Like me, something happened to her physical constitution as she approached her thirtieth year, and she finally broke down and committed the one unpardonable sin for a woman of her class during the Great Depression: she hired a nanny. Growing up, my mother's recurring stories about this stressed what a drastic measure it was to have paid domestic help at that time. "Not a single person your grandmother knew hired nannies or maids," my mother told me repeatedly, but always as if it were for the first time. "She wasn't working, and as far as most people were concerned, she wasn't sick. So hiring someone to come in and change diapers and wash the floors seemed crazy. It really was a bold and extravagant move back then."

Although my grandmother didn't talk about it much with me, I imagine having to hire help was a shock for her also. Up until then, she'd singlehandedly ensured her mighty backyard garden was planted, maintained, and harvested. Her basement cellar was perpetually stocked with enough canned carrots, beets, and pickles to get the family through the brutally cold winters. At all times she could be counted on to be there for aging parents and grandparents and struggling neighbors. With very little help from her husband, her four children had been fed and cared for and always had everything they needed.

And then, on the cusp of middle age, she found herself unable to complete even the simplest of tasks. Without much warning, the endless cycle of dishes and laundry that was the burden of most women of this era suddenly overwhelmed my grandmother. "Eating took too much effort," my mother would lament. "Even fastening her apron was a chore."

The second member of my family to be incapacitated by the family curse was my mother. She was a force to be reckoned with before she got sick. Despite working two jobs, she managed to cart me around to dance classes and gymnastics lessons, cook evening dinners with my father, and spend time socializing with family and friends — all the while staying on top of the rigorous cleaning schedule she'd devised for our home. She could spend evenings at the local pool splashing around with her nieces, clap enthusiastically from the sidelines at every recital and meet, and host humble yet love-filled dinner parties for her closest family members and friends. But no matter how many cups of coffee she would share with her favorite cousin or her cherished brother, without fail the walls, curtains, cupboards, and floorboards were meticulously cleaned according to that timetable. Life moved at a fast pace with my mother, and everyone around her had better keep up.

But despite her formidable energy, when my mother was about thirty years old her body started changing in ways that hampered her breakneck pace. With the emerging sleepless nights and plummeting energy levels, her morning alarm clock was suddenly met with despair. Once at work, the basic filing and scheduling requirements of her secretarial job — tasks that intellectually were previously far beneath her — now took everything she had. On weekends her persistent body aches kept her from being able to sit long enough to finish making her prized macramé and paper tole projects, and although she still made sure she did it, carting me to my swim lessons had unfortunately become an exhausting chore.

It was as if she had . . . the flu. Sort of. But not really. She had some flu-like symptoms some of the time. But none of the symptoms all of the time. This was a clever and sneaky adversary, popping its head up just long enough to cause problems and then disappearing just long enough to make it appear as if nothing were wrong.

Within a year, vacations were no longer even on my family's radar, and my mother's mysterious ailments forced her to quit her job. And because her response to the question *Are you feeling any better yet?* was always met by a firm *No,* by that time most of her friends had also disappeared. It seems bystanders don't have much endurance for the in-between. She wasn't cheery, she never had good news, and people got tired of hearing it. The unspoken message she consistently heard was that she'd better get busy living or get busy dying.

Keeping with family tradition, it all started for me shortly before I turned thirty years old. And despite knowing what both my mother and grandmother had already gone through at this exact age, when it happened to me, I somehow really just thought I had the flu.

At the last minute, my husband and I discovered that a friend's destination wedding in Mexico would be scheduled to take place immediately after we were set to return from a month-long dream vacation we'd booked in Western Europe. And since we were not wanting or willing to miss out on either trip, we somehow managed to find a way to pull off both.

One morning about three weeks into our European adventure, while lying in the guesthouse bed staring at the ceiling, I realized that I absolutely could not get up. I was in Paris — PARIS — for the first time in my life, and I couldn't muster the energy to leave the four walls surrounding me to even stumble out to a café and grab a bite of *petit déjeuner*. My mind felt dull and groggy, and my body ached all over. Despite how desperate I was to saunter through the Louvre and peruse the shops on Champs-Élysées, there was no denying that for the remainder of that day, I was trapped in that room.

I had no right to complain. The rest of that European expedition along with the subsequent party-filled Mexican nuptial celebrations went off without a hitch. Of those forty-five or so total days spent abroad, forty-four of them were filled with twelve-hour days of balls-to-the-wall sightseeing and exploring. I'd set off on these holidays toting a thick binder filled with activities planned for every single place we were to visit. (I'm a planner, through and through, and this trait of mine doesn't ever take a break — not even when I'm on vacation.) Of those forty-five days that we were gone, this one day in Paris was the only day of rest that I felt I needed. And given that I bounced back from that day to continue on our journey, I didn't give it a second thought.

Our six weeks of escapades spanning seven different countries eventually wrapped up, and reluctantly we boarded our final flight to head back to The Real World. By the time we finally walked in the door of our beloved house, it was after midnight. Collapsing in bed, there was no time to process how I felt, or even what I might manage to find to eat for breakfast the next morning.

With no remaining vacation days from my full-time job left, I had to go straight back to work the day after these back-to-back trips were over. My first morning home consisted of dragging my dog-tired self out of bed and groggily getting myself off to work. It was a rough start to the day, but I'd expected that. I was certain that, once I got going, my puffy face and bloodshot eyes would fade, and I'd get back into the swing of things in no time. Because in my experience, there was just no way to remain in this dulled down state while dealing with the challenging demands of being a social worker. But as I pushed myself to attend rounds and meet with the families of the fragile infant inpatients on the busy neonatal intensive care unit that I worked on, I was not perking up — at all. The dizziness I felt when I stood up often forced me to find the closest object on which to brace myself to keep from falling over. Normally I took the stairs while at work, but on this day the elevator was the only feasible option. It was as if low doses of poison were running through my veins, with waves of nausea hitting me at unexpected intervals. I couldn't eat, and the coffee I was guzzling wasn't improving things for me one bit.

I assumed it was the flu. I was run down, I worked in a hospital full of sick people, and it was flu season, so having the flu made perfect sense. I can only imagine what my boss and coworkers were thinking when I proceeded to go home sick after just haven taken so much vacation time. Being a social worker in a busy inner-city hospital, I'm sure my absence was felt. But whatever this was had leveled me, and I had no choice but to stay home for a few days to rest and try to recover.

If this was the flu, then this one was serious business. During those first few days, as my alarm rang, I'd wake up and quickly realize that the venom occupying my cells still remained. With each passing day, I'd reluctantly admit that even if my life depended on it I couldn't yet drag myself back to work. It was one full week before this beast of an illness eased up enough to allow me to return to my job. Calling in sick that first day was stressful; having that conversation with my boss five days in a row was crippling. I hated feeling like such an unreliable coworker, but I'd had no choice but to stay home until I recovered.

After this full week off from work sick, back to work I went. My boss rejoiced (or at least decided to hold off on firing me), and all was right in the world again.

Or not. I was only able to manage a few more days back at work before the poison in my veins started to return. I honestly had no idea what was going on. *Was this another flu? Or the same one — that had somehow come back?* Whatever was going on, I was sick again and, to my horror, needed to take even more time off work.

Each time I spent a day or two more at home resting, I'd feel a bit more energized and head back to work. I'd assume that this was all finally behind me and that the determined flu that had been plaguing me was at long last gone. But once back at work, without fail, by the time lunch rolled around it would take everything I had to keep going. Sometimes, in my small closet of an office, I'd even brush my paperwork to the side and curl up on top of my desk and try to take a nap. When someone inevitably knocked on my door I'd jump up, fluff my hair, plaster an energetic smile on my face, and pretend that, instead of sleeping, I'd just been interrupted from some important task on my computer.

I'd cringe every time my work pager's beep beckoned me to consult on a new case, because although physically I was definitely struggling, an even bigger hurdle was the attempt to function mentally. My brain was steeped in a thick fog, and my memory was significantly impaired. Whenever I had to talk to patients or doctors, I felt as though I were putting on an act. *Just look confident*, I'd tell myself. *Say some big words, and no one will notice that your head right now is actually an empty shell.*

At home, dinner transformed from hot meals enjoyed at the kitchen table to protein shakes quickly whipped up in the blender and consumed from the couch. Despite my workouts historically always being a priority, I no longer even dreamed about trying to get to the gym. My laundry piled up, and my work clothes went un-ironed. I'd always lived for the weekends, but now instead of looking forward to the Saturday-night dinner parties and nights out with friends, I counted down to the weekends so that I could enjoy two full guilt-free days of rest.

Worst of all was the toll the illness took on my marriage. I was the life of the party, and I suspect that *being fun* had always been one of my biggest draws for my husband. Now I just cried — a lot. I yelled at him words of frustration meant for this mysterious illness. I looked at him daily with intense desperation in my eyes that begged him to somehow magically make all my pain and suffering stop. Gone were the lighthearted chats about what mischievous antics our friends and relatives were up to. Now all I talked about was how frustrated and confused and sick I was. I bailed on every single invitation to hang out with our friends. Aside from his consoling hugs to soak up my tears, I denied every single one of his touches.

I was a wreck, and I wasn't getting any better.

As most people do, when I was first got sick I tried to gut it out, but it was to no avail. After all, there's not much you can do for the flu except let it run its course. But when I couldn't shake it by the third week I decided to visit my family doctor. Although I'd never actually gone to see her for anything that serious before (I think the worst was to experiment with various birth control pills to see which had the least adverse side-effects), when I did come in I'd always liked her and respected her treatment approach. She was friendly and had been helpful in the past, and I felt good about having her in my corner. I was sure she would be able to tell me what was wrong and, moreover, patch me up in no time.

"I've been sick lately," I started off tentatively, trying to figure out how to concisely sum up weeks' worth of suffering into a couple of sentences. "I got the flu a while back, and it just won't go away."

As she looked at me in that supportive way that she always did, I immediately started to feel reassured that everything would be ok. "It's probably just a persistent flu," she said. "There's a bad one going around that lots of people have been struggling with. But let's run some tests to make sure it isn't something else."

She performed the routine lab tests you'd expect her to do, and I dutifully filled up vial after vial of blood and threw in a urine sample for good measure. Everything was fine and going exactly as I had imagined it would — until all the tests came back normal. According to the lab, I was perfectly fine. She sent me off with a prescription for ample fluids and lots of rest and assured me that soon life would return back to normal.

It didn't. I didn't get better. If anything I started to get worse. And feeling worse, I kept coming back. But there were no more tests left to run, and yet I kept appearing in her office. Not being a doctor I had no idea how to proceed — that was her specialty. What *was* my responsibility was to figure out how, despite my persistent absences, I was going to keep my job.

"I was wondering if you could sign some paperwork for my employer that would allow me to reduce my hours for the next few weeks," I hesitantly squeaked out. "I can't keep up with my job and I'm out of sick leave, so until we figure this out, I really need to take a bit of time off."

As I sat in her office on her vinyl patient's table covered in that white roll-out paper — a seat that on its own somehow always makes you feel sick and vulnerable — I watched as she asked, with an incredulous look on her face, "How am I supposed to sign paperwork for you to be off work when there is nothing wrong with you?"

Her response shattered me. If there was one person who I thought knew I was sick — really sick — it was my doctor. She was going to be my savior, my lifeline, the one person who could help me through this and make sure things turned out ok. And now her words said that the fact that I could barely get out of bed most days was irrelevant. I felt hurt and betrayed, but I also felt embarrassed. She really thought that I was faking this, trying to scam the system by outright lying. I quickly gathered my things and left the office, never to see her again.

We like to make fun of people who Google symptoms and self-diagnose, and of course, this can lead to dangerous and even reckless behavior. But after what I experienced I have nothing but respect for people who take the wheel and start steering the direction of their treatment. The vital lesson I learned that day in my family doctor's office was that I needed to take charge and put the health of my body into my own hands.

Let me be clear: in no way do I think that doing your own research should replace consultations with licensed healthcare practitioners. Without a doubt, we still need doctors — good doctors. They have both knowledge and practical training that would be near impossible to obtain on our own. But we also need doctors who listen to their patients and don't treat them as the sum total of their lab results, who see the whole person and not just the symptoms.

In my case, the eventual result of that visit was actually quite liberating. I would no longer trust doctors to be my single source of truth. I would no longer rely on them for all my answers, and I would no longer assume that everything they told me was correct. I would get second and third opinions. I would do my own research. I would dig and I would question and I would analyze until my diagnosis and my treatment plan fit how I was actually feeling — not what a lab report said.

Since the standard tests my doctor administered had come up empty, I started to look elsewhere for answers. From my research, I learned that even from Canada I could make use of some specialized medical labs in the United States that (for a price) could provide me with a more comprehensive picture of what was happening in my body. At the time I couldn't have cared less about the cost — I just wanted answers. In fact, the large price tag was actually a bit alluring. If the tests cost that much, I figured they must be good.

I contacted one such American lab and was given a list of

local private doctors who could order the tests for me — the closest doctor being a six-hour round trip from my house. But I would not be deterred, and I promptly booked an appointment with him. And with that began my official introduction to the two-tiered medical system in Canada that of which I'd been completely unaware.

As a Canadian citizen with access to our universal healthcare system, I was fortunate in that I'd never directly paid for healthcare services before in my life. Until that point, I didn't even know that private medical clinics existed in my country. Although I appreciated so many things about universal healthcare, I quickly started to recognize some of the benefits of going the private route. For example, when doctors have to compete for your business, they might try a little harder to be a better doctor to you. And if exceptional doctors can charge more, the incentives are even greater for them to do great work. For better or worse, once healthcare becomes a business, private physicians are incentivized to provide better care and work harder to earn your business. There are of course downfalls to this approach, but at that point in time I only experienced the perks.

Immediately this new clinic filled me with hope. Instead of a cramped and noisy waiting room filled with wailing toddlers and wheezing seniors, this doctor's office offered up a reception area where a small trickling waterfall sent soothing sounds reverberating off the large windows that invited in ample warm and natural light. As I sat on the plush waiting room sofa and filled out my details on the papers attached to the clipboard I'd been handed, I noticed that on the coffee table in front of me was a large three-ring binder filled with success stories and thank-you letters from past patients of this clinic that someone had compiled and preserved neatly in plastic sleeves. This was definitely an improvement from the random coffee-table magazines with pages stuck together — the germ-covered weapons of biological warfare typical of most medical clinics that I was used to. These stories in this binder were inspiring and lent credibility to this doctor that I'd yet to even meet, and I immediately began to fantasize about what my own contribution to this binder might be. Before I had even set foot in his office, I could clearly envision myself healed and singing the praises of this remarkable place.

Just as I had with the waiting room, I liked Dr. M. right from the start. His exotic and intoxicating accent (which I'd later learn was South African) gave him an air of possessing prized knowledge that I felt the unexciting Canadian-born doctors I was used to seeing could not possibly possess. And more importantly, he seemed as if he actually believed me when I said I was sick, and he appeared committed to helping me get to the bottom of whatever was causing my illness. What also really interested me was his Integrative Medicine philosophy that combined Western and alternative approaches to medicine in a collaborative process with the patient. Everything about this new doctor and his glorious healing center seemed contrary to the public medical system to which I was accustomed — the one that, in the first time I truly needed it, had failed me so completely.

Before this day, I don't think I'd ever spent more than five or ten minutes in a doctor's office at one time. So it was much to my astonishment when this first appointment with Dr. M. lasted over *two hours*. From lab work to symptom inventories to personality tests to detailed family histories, we covered it all. By the time I was preparing to leave that office, he knew what I ate, what kind of flooring was in my house, and how often I had sex.

As we talked about the struggles of the women of my family before me, I could see the unease and consternation building in his eyes. As far as I was concerned, I was in his office for what I suspected would be a pricey but hopefully relatively quick fix. I wanted to hear that I had a B-12 deficiency or that the mold in my potted plants was what had been causing all this fuss in my life.

He could see I didn't want to hear it. And I could tell he didn't want to say it. But it seemed there was no way around it. So after an incredibly long and awkward pause, my new esteemed doctor slowly exhaled before saying the words I'd spent most of my life determined not to hear.

"I think you have chronic fatigue syndrome."

2

ACCEPTING THE DIAGNOSIS

When I got sick I really had no idea what was going on, despite all the signs being there. I feel a tad foolish now for not having seen them for what they truly were. Even before my first CFS symptom, with my family history, I should have known what was likely to come. But my head was planted firmly in the sand, my denial irrefutable.

My diagnosis of chronic fatigue syndrome felt like a death sentence, and I don't think that anything could've prepared me for the total devastation that this brought to my life. This illness seemed to instantly strip away virtually everything that I loved. My hopes for the future were likewise mostly gone. It was like I'd fallen asleep and woken up in a parallel universe. Almost overnight, every single moment of every single day was irreversibly changed. In what felt like the blink of an eye, my life transformed from being incredible, or at the very least solidly average, to the stuff of nightmares.

This sickness, this *flu*, ended up lasting over ten years. *Ten fucking years.*

But time was the least of what I lost.

If I'd truly appreciated how tough those upcoming years were going to be, I don't think I would've initially cared quite so much about the shape of my ass. But acceptance of CFS for me came in stages, and those were still the early days.

It was always buried deep somewhere in the back of my mind that this *could* happen to me, but honestly, for whatever reason, I was mostly convinced that it wouldn't. I had always felt like such a different person than my mother. I didn't think that I looked like her, and I felt that our personalities were very different. And somehow, as unbelievable as it might sound, these differences made me feel somehow immune to CFS. I assumed that we had dramatically different genetic makeups and that, because of this, I would be ok.

Writing these words now I see how ridiculous that is. But denial is a powerful force. To admit that there might be a genetic component to CFS that I had inherited was to admit that at any moment my life could be stolen from me. I think that when faced with the choice of living a life in fear of getting sick, versus a life of deluding myself, the latter was just easier. I simply *decided* that it would never happen to me, as if it was somehow that easy. I was so active and I had such a busy life that it seemed impossible that anything could ever slow me down. Maybe, if I constantly kept moving, I could never be stopped. Once you slow down, that's when they get you. *Right?*

It was probably better to not see it coming. This meant that I'd gotten to enjoy my healthy years relatively worry-free. There was very little information on CFS during my mother's time with this disease that could have helped me prevent it in myself, so whether I knew it was coming or not probably wouldn't have mattered.

My grandmother didn't even have the benefit of a diagnosis. What doctors my grandmother managed to see were not able to tell her much. Back then only basic medical procedures were covered by the Canadian healthcare system — and certainly not to investigate what was lightly dismissed as just "being run down" in the parlance of the day. Nor would the meager allowance that my grandfather (a somewhat unfeeling and pragmatic man) set aside from the family's finances cover anything but the most rudimentary of explorations into my grandmother's medical condition. The doctors that she did manage to see left her with the impression that any efforts at getting better were futile. "This is just how you are built," one well-meaning physician had told her after one examination. "You are a pony, not a horse, and you will just have to find a way to live like this."

Despite it being decades after her own mother's health complications, my mother faced much of the same confusion and dead ends. "It's your hormones," one overly confident and quick-to-diagnose doctor initially informed her. "You're going to need a hysterectomy if you ever want to feel better." So, without hesitation, my overly trusting and desperate mother proceeded to undergo major surgery and have her uterus removed — only to not feel one iota better afterward.

As time went on her illness persisted, and more and more tests came back normal. Before long it didn't seem to matter how many doctors she saw; the conclusion was always that she was depressed. "Of course I'm depressed!" my mother would cry out in frustration. "I'm depressed *because* of this illness!"

But instead of receiving a diagnosis from these doctors or, at the very least, some form of a label that would describe the sudden and perplexing set of symptoms that had ground her life to a screeching halt, all she was sent off with was an endless array of prescriptions for antidepressants.

I'd be lying if I didn't admit that I was depressed when I heard the words chronic fatigue syndrome. The words themselves speak to just how pessimistic a diagnosis it is — you don't get better from something that's *chronic*, and *syndrome* just implied medical confusion.

Yet even with the knowledge of what my grandmother and mother went through, I really didn't know at the time of getting my diagnosis just how hard it would be to learn how to live with this illness. When I heard those words it just felt like it was more than I could handle. I was suffering so much, and I was so scared by what was happening to my body. It was so confusing and terrifying that I wouldn't have wished the experience on my worst enemy. And yet I can look back on those first days of the diagnosis and recognize that they were relatively easy. I hadn't been living with CFS for that long and had no idea of how many long days were ahead of me.

With CFS, every single moment of every single day felt difficult to get through. And since I didn't even really understand myself what was happening to me, explaining it to others felt nearly impossible. It all seemed so vague and yet so severe, and I completely lacked the vocabulary for it. Whatever was happening was way beyond feeling fatigued or tired. *Tired* I could push through. Whatever this was, there was no pushing through it. It felt as if all the cells in my body were suddenly made out of lead. I felt like a prisoner in my own body.

Just getting through even one day could feel like a marathon. I felt physically changed hour by hour and even minute by minute. Every bite of food I put into my mouth still seemed to make me feel worse. Bouts of nausea and rounds of headaches seemed to come and go at will, and thinking clearly and being able to remember the simplest of things could feel impossible. The exertion required to socialize, for even just a simple conversation with a friend, could drain what little energy reserves I had and completely finish me off.

Of course, most of those first days were days where I would most likely be alone and talk to no one. A day where I might not get out of the same pajamas I'd already been wearing for days. Where I'd check my email ten times just to feel some sort of connection to the world. Where I'd reluctantly finish off another great book, but since it'd be one of a hundred I'd already read that year I'd have trouble appreciating it. A day where at some point I might cry, where I might beg the universe for a break, for strength, or for just a little help. A day where I felt that not a single soul on the planet knew how I felt, and if they did, then they'd likely be isolated too, and I'd have no hope of finding them.

These were days where, when I could actually manage to get out of bed, I'd have nothing to distract myself from my ridiculous anxiety about the chairs being straight and things being put away. Where walking to the corner of my block, on the rare days that I could manage it, felt like a vacation. Where I'd probably buy something online that I absolutely could not afford, just to feel one moment of happiness, escape, and distraction from all that was wrong and all that was missing. Of watching the world go by, go on, as if without me.

It was without a doubt the scariest and most difficult thing I had ever gone through.

Even though I of course knew that horrible things happened to people all the time, much of them far worse than what was happening to me, I still struggled to come to terms with the injustice of it all. At the time I really thought that the whole situation was really unfair. I'm not sure why I felt that I was so special, why I alone should be able to evade life's major struggles, but I did.

As far as I was concerned, my life had been stolen from me. I felt as if the city that I lived in (hell, maybe the whole country) should come to a screeching halt so that we could all band together and figure out how to save me from this nightmare. It sounds a bit crazy to me now, but it's really how I felt.

Until that point in time I'd lived a mostly happy, healthy, and privileged life, so when a dose of turmoil came my way it hit me hard. The definition of a hard life is not absolute, and my past version of one definitely loses its impact when compared to the version that far too many others live today. In this world there are so many people that experience more challenges in one single day than what I've experienced in my entire worst year. Perhaps I'd had no right to complain and little right to feel sorry for myself. Yes, it's true, another person's suffering or situation does not and should not diminish our own, but with the clarity of hindsight I can't help but feel a little guilty over the tantrums and pity parties that were the norm for me then. I'd never dream of judging another CFS sufferer for indulging in these feelings and would be most understanding of why they were feeling that way, but as I suspect is typical for many of us, I am by far the harshest when it comes to judging myself.

In time, I slowly got over that feeling of injustice. I came to realize and accept that we all have our crosses to bear (many of us more than one). I wasn't special or immune. I learned to take this challenge and use it to strengthen me and shape me into something better than I was before. It would be a while before I would get to that place, but eventually, I did.

Despite whatever acceptance of this illness I gained, it's still sometimes difficult for me, even now, to think or talk about it. When CFS was at its worst it could take me to some really dark places. My quality of life often felt so low, and my days such a battle, that I really struggled to cope with it all. I knew that all my stress and depression were making the CFS symptoms worse, but I had no idea how to cope with things any better than I was. It was like trying to learn how to be at peace with my jailer.

I also felt so incredibly alone in my experience. Despite people's best efforts, I'm certain absolutely no one in my world understood what I was going through. Thanks to my first doctor, I spent a lot of time worrying that people thought that I was making up this whole experience or, at the very least, significantly exaggerating it all. I think it can be hard for people to understand and believe in an invisible illness like CFS. I didn't look any different. I didn't sound any different. I wasn't even receiving any sort of recognized or standardized treatment. Yet there I was, claiming to be almost completely debilitated.

For the most part, life with CFS was a really confusing experience for me. My body was telling me to do nothing but rest, but somehow my mind struggled to get on board. For a long time, that all-powerful mind-body connection seemed to be having a major disconnect. I wasn't used to sitting still for very long, and the adjustment to an almost completely sedentary way of life was definitely a challenging one.

I also never really knew how any day was going to go, which served to intensify that unbearable feeling of being out of control. Some days I woke up feeling really rough but would start to feel a tad better as the day went on. Other days I started out feeling relatively good but would then slowly deteriorate. Some days were just bad start to finish. There was never — not once — a day where I simply felt good.

There was *one* thing that was fairly predictable, which was that after any kind of mental or physical exertion, I would feel completely depleted. I couldn't seem to recover from any form of exercise or physical activity. And as time went on, the amount of exertion required to lay me out was less and less. The smallest of activities could take days, or even weeks, from which to recover. All I seemed to feel like doing was rest, but regardless of how much rest I got, I never felt any better.

My brain was also hit hard by CFS. For a while, my thinking was so foggy that if I went anywhere in my house to do anything, I'd have to take a note with me telling me what to do when I got there. I felt ridiculous wandering around my house with reminders on Post-it notes stuck to my fingers, but it was the only way I could ever remember why I'd gotten up and walked to another room in the first place. It wasn't that, on occasion, I might forget once I got there — it was that I most definitely would, every single time.

I hardly ever got out of bed or off of the couch, nothing in my body seemed to be working as it should, and everything in my life seemed to be falling apart.

For a long time, my CFS diagnosis felt completely useless. It didn't shed any light on the cause of this disease or offer any insight into a prognosis or treatment. Diagnosis is purely symptom-based, and both doctors and the scientific literature alike mostly come up empty when tasked with explaining in any meaningful way what is happening with this illness. The label of CFS didn't seem to actually mean anything and I felt served as nothing more than a pointless descriptive label for my particular set of symptoms.

I even thought that the name *chronic fatigue syndrome* was terrible. It's an injustice to CFS sufferers to give it such a blasé name. What I and the women in my family before me went through was so much more and so much worse than *fatigue*. The name makes it sound like the people who have it *maybe get a little tired once in a while*. It's the type of name that invokes some well-meaning healthy people, upon hearing it, to respond with infuriating sentiments like *I know what you mean, I get tired sometimes too*. It's like those t-shirts: my life had been completely stripped away from me and all I got was a lousy explanation called *chronic fatigue*. I used to joke that whoever named this condition might as well have named it *crazy lazy syndrome* because that sounded about equally as reputable.

I'm pretty sure that a cancer diagnosis would've made me feel less helpless than facing CFS did. I in no way mean to downplay the seriousness of cancer, and its comparison to CFS is probably an insult to cancer victims. The "c" word absolutely terrifies me, and logically speaking, I have no doubt that cancer can be a much tougher diagnosis to deal with than CFS. But after having watched what my grandmother and then my mother went through, logic wasn't really a part of the equation for me anymore. I'd seen firsthand what CFS could do, and it absolutely terrified me.

But this was the only diagnosis I was going to get, so I started to make what peace with it I could.

Before I got sick, I believed that indulging in any kind of downtime was tantamount to being lazy. I often had two jobs, one full-time job as a social worker as well as a side hustle of some sort where I worked evenings and weekends in a restaurant or a bar. On top of this, I was often enrolled in part-time or full-time university courses as well. I was also quite sociable when I wasn't working, going out with friends to restaurants, bars, and parties and staying out into the wee hours of the morning. Add to this the five to six days per week that I went to the gym, sometimes even twice in one day, and my schedule was more than a little packed.

At the time, I was so unbelievably proud of how hard I worked and how busy I was. These were *definite* points of pride for me. Back then the glorification of being busy was all the rage, so it was difficult for me to see the harm in this toxic mindset. Virtually everyone I knew prided themselves on how busy they were, which made it much easier for me to wear my own habit of running myself into the ground like a badge of honor.

In hindsight I see that, for me, this attempt at overachieving was, for the most part, a result of my low self-esteem. I thought that if I worked hard enough, was educated enough, had a fit enough body, a fancy enough house, and enough friends, I might finally feel like a worthwhile human being.

It's heartbreaking now to think about how hard I was on myself back then. I had so much to prove, to no one in particular, and I would stop at almost nothing to achieve my goals. And despite my best efforts, I was still pretty clueless about life, so unfortunately much of my toiling was often in vain. All my hard work certainly hadn't made me the picture of good health and success that I desired to be. But I tried. Relentlessly, I tried.

I remember one day, years before CFS set in, when my husband and I moved into our first home together. It was a modest two-bedroom duplex that we'd just finished renovating. It was a humble space, but this was the first place in my life that I'd owned, so I was radiating pride. After the renovations were complete, the newly laid floor tiles and walls of fresh paint eagerly awaited our arrival, and I was beyond excited to get our lives started together there.

I was determined to completely unpack every single one of our boxes on the first day. I was uncomfortable with any kind of disorder, and so I wanted everything put away immediately in its new place. I wanted Day One of Our New Life Together to begin perfectly the very next morning, with our home superbly organized and everything ready to go.

My impatience and stubbornness had me unpacking and organizing for hours on end. By about midnight on that first day in our new home, my body was screaming at me for rest. I really felt that, despite being so determined to get everything finished, physically I just couldn't do any more.

But instead of stopping and going to bed, I decided that my mind was more powerful than my body and that I would use my sheer will to push past whatever limits my body was attempting to impose on me. I continued to work until everything was completely unpacked, and I remember silently (and somewhat flippantly) thinking, *I wonder what happens when you push way past your limits? Well, I guess I'm about to find out!*

I clearly didn't really think anything that bad would come from working past my limits, otherwise I like to think that I would've had the good sense to pause my unpacking efforts and go to bed. It's mind-boggling now to think how completely naive I was then to the effects of not taking care of myself. Well into my twenties I still had that feeling of invincibility that I suspect most people wisely leave behind in their teens. Listening to my body was a completely foreign concept to me, even when my body was screaming bloody murder.

I pushed this hard in absolutely single every area of my life, with rarely a thought about what toll this strain might take on my body or mind. It really never occurred to me that there might be a cost. I seemed content to float through life in a bit of a haze, rarely pausing long enough to look too closely at what was going on around me. *Do more, work harder, and don't question much* seemed to be my life's philosophy.

In retrospect, it's not surprising that my health eventually crashed in spectacular fashion. I'm not saying that getting CFS was my fault. But I do think that I had created the perfect conditions for it to take hold of me and shut me up in its prison. I wasn't taking care of myself or treating my body well, and I now understand that that sort of behavior comes at a price. Despite probably having a genetic predisposition to getting CFS, had I taken better care of myself, perhaps I might never have even gotten it.

What *is* still a bit surprising to me is how quickly it all fell apart for me, how fast the regression from health to sickness took place. It was like a rug — that I didn't even know was there and was so vital to my functioning — was suddenly pulled out from under me, leaving me flailing and confused and incredibly sick.

Looking back I often think about what I would tell that terrified woman exiting Dr. M.'s office. The most important thing I would tell her — the thing that I would make her sit down on the front stoop and hear again and again until she could repeat it to me verbatim — is that no matter how bad CFS was, it would be *up to me* how bad it would actually be. I would tell her that although I'd gotten some of the same symptoms as my mother and grandmother, genetics are not destiny. I would tell her that my choices — what I chose to do with my body — is what would determine my prognosis.

Nothing was set. This wasn't a death sentence. My life wasn't doomed.

I'd tell myself that after I exited Dr. M.'s office, before I even got in my car, I should make an appointment with a counselor — because before I could ever have any hope of strengthening my body, I absolutely had to make myself mentally strong first. I most certainly was not equipped to deal with this all by myself, and my friends and family, although superb, were not equipped to deal with all this either (and it absolutely would not be fair to put all of this on them even if they were). I would tell me that with CFS I had a formidable opponent in front of me, and I needed to absolutely have my head in the game. Initially, I could allow myself to take a beating and feel sorry for myself for a short time, but I wasn't to get trapped there.

I would tell myself to just feel the anger and devastation and pain course through my veins, and then let it drain out of my body for good. Perspective is everything, and as impossible as it might feel, my ability to immediately start finding the good in all of this is what would serve me best.

I would stress to me then that another key to accepting and surviving this diagnosis would be to, as fast as I could, find others who were going through the same thing. There is nothing more soothing or more healing than being able to look in the eyes of someone who knows what your particular kind of hell feels like. That this connection to people facing this same hell could be my lifeline as I searched for my own path out of this.

And lastly, I'd tell myself not to be ashamed of this diagnosis. That this is a legitimate and debilitating condition that devastates many unsuspecting victims. To own it and not to hide from it. When people ask you what is wrong with you — hold your head up high as you say it aloud:

"I have chronic fatigue syndrome."

II

LIVING WITH SHACKLES

3

SIFTING THROUGH SNAKE OIL

Dr. M. became my healing guru and I his model patient, complying with absolutely everything he told me to do down to the letter. But doing so required single-minded dedication, and I was truly relieved when, with Dr. M.'s assistance, I was able to take a medical leave of absence from my job. It started as just a couple months, but when all the extensions were said and done, I was off work for a total of eighteen months.

Dr. M. was a spectacular doctor, but he was not cheap. It cost me thousands of dollars per month to keep up with the costs of the appointments, lab tests, and supplements he prescribed. My supplement bill alone ran me about two thousand Canadian dollars per month. It was expensive, but I didn't care. I was mailing every bodily fluid I had to various American labs and got back enough detailed results to fill the four-inch binder I'd bought in which to save all my test results. I was going broke (and not slowly), but I was thrilled nevertheless. I had to get my life back, and to me, having a professional working so hard to help me do that was priceless.

My strong, confident, and determined mother, having no such diagnosis nor doctor in her corner, set off in search of her own solutions. This being the early eighties, finding information meant doing a lot of leg work. There would be no absent-minded clicking through websites from the comfort of her home while sipping on a latte. No one had a YouTube channel devoted to remedying chronic fatigue, and there was certainly no way to jump in on the latest Twitter debate on the subject.

In this pre-digital world, when your doctor didn't have answers, you went to the library. This was my mother, so it took her less than a month to exhaust everything they had there that might assist her. When trips to other local public libraries came up short, my mother, who'd herself never before set foot in a university, sat herself down amongst the fresh-faced college students at the city's biggest university library and searched through what academia had to offer.

But even there she found nothing.

Going off the advice of well-meaning friends and relatives, she sought out naturopathic doctors and tried various supposed vitamin cures. She endured acupuncture sessions complete with electrical probes meant to find the imbalances in the invisible energy pathways in her body. She consulted mysterious "physicians" that had her clasp assorted glass vials while they "measured" her body's responses to each and determined her cure. An elderly man in a small herbal shop in Chinatown once sent her off with bags of roots she was to boil before drinking their repugnant broth. She'd come home from some appointments sporting cylindrical hickeys all over her body, the result of sessions where some therapist had put flammable liquid inside glass cups, set it on fire, and then suctioned the smoking cups all over her body.

Nothing helped. But as she would say, *when you're desperate and the doctors aren't doing anything, you try whatever you can.*

Little did I know to what extent I would embrace her outlook — even with doctors on my side. During those first two years, I was a living, breathing, healing plan in action. Virtually every thought, ounce of energy, and penny I had went into my trying to get better. After witnessing what my mother and grandmother went through, I knew that a life that included CFS wasn't going to be for me. I just wasn't up for that. I just couldn't, *wouldn't* live that way. I wish I could say that I was a stronger person and better able to make lemonade from life's lemons, but this illness made me horribly depressed. I knew it was either beat CFS or else I might just give up on living. So keep spending I did.

Like my mother, I too read everything in sight about my condition. Dr. M. encouraged me in this regard and (within reason) to experiment with anything that I thought might help. He wanted me to educate myself and play an active role in my recovery, and I often walked out of my appointments with him with a list of recommended reading on various topics related to my condition. It was awesome to feel like I was taking control.

My thirst for health-related information was insatiable, and I devoured books by the dozens. With seemingly endless days spent laid out on the couch or in bed, there was no shortage of opportunity for me to read. Aside from the occasional light read about vampires or shopaholics to distract me and keep me sane, the bulk of what I read was focused on the information out there that might be able to get me better. I plowed through books on nutrition, exercise, and anything that had the word *fatigue* in the title. I also read books that focused on healing from diseases other than CFS, just in case they might contain some nuggets of information that could be helpful for healing my condition as well. The wackiest book I read suggested that the key to healing was eating one small boiled potato before bed. It didn't matter; I was absolutely determined to get well, and I consumed every piece of health-related information I could possibly get my hands on (and of course that potato as well).

Since the world of Western medicine didn't seem to be putting out much in terms of books on CFS at the time, I dove headfirst into the literary world of holistic and alternative medicine. I found it fascinating to learn about all the ways that I could naturally support my body's health through simple acts such as consuming juiced turnip tops while soaking in a bath of Epsom salts. I liked the idea of being on the same team as my body and loved finding ways to help it do what it was innately built to do.

However, I quickly learned that not everything I read was backed by rigorous scientific research. In fact, much of what I read didn't appear to be backed by any sort of research at all. For all I knew I could've been sifting through a sea of nothing but snake oil. But that didn't deter me. I was desperate to heal, so I soaked up as much information (and Epsom salts) as I could, scientifically backed or otherwise, in hopes that alternative medicine might be excelling in CFS treatment in the ways that Western medicine seemed to be lacking.

Although some of what I read definitely sounded like nonsense, I actually found many of these holistic health books quite convincing. The world of alternative healing boasted

unbiased treatment options, free from the influence of pharmaceutical companies or any other parties whose sole motivation
might simply be to make a profit. *Of course* no one was aware of
the potential healing effects of oranges or the sun, because
these things couldn't be patented. Since no one could restrict
access to them or get rich off their healing powers, no one with
any far-reaching platform was actively promoting their benefits.

The more I read, the more convinced I became that the
keys to health I sought might be easily and cheaply available in
nature, just waiting to be utilized. Alternative medicine really
felt like it had everything I had been searching for. It explained
why doctors focusing solely on Western medicine couldn't help
me, and it gave me hope that with the help of integrative physicians like Dr. M. I could still be cured. Everything about it just
felt right, so I jumped in headfirst and consumed every single
bit of information I could find.

Virtually every single treatment I read about in every single
book was supposedly vital for healing. Modalities such as chro-
motherapy, inclined bed therapy, and rife frequency tech-
nology were advocated repeatedly in scores of different books,
somehow lending these therapies credence through their repetition, and making them seem all the more essential to wellness.
Having only so much energy to spare, hours to fill, and dollars
to spend made it quite challenging for me to filter out what I
should try and what I could safely ignore.

Through my research, I also became convinced that I had a
whole slew of health conditions in addition to CFS. Or perhaps
these were underlying conditions that were actually the cause
of the CFS? Or possibly they were a result of it? Whether these
ailments were co-morbidities or came as a package deal, I really

wasn't sure. But as long as I fixed them all, the distinction really didn't matter to me.

It's uncanny how the longer my list of afflictions became, the easier time I had of dealing with it all. This long list served to break down the issues in my body into more specific, manageable, and more easily treatable chunks. And at least to me, my health problems also started to become more legitimate sounding. CFS alone might not sound sufficient to cause such devastation in my life, but my new laundry list of ailments did.

Regardless of whether these health issues were real or imagined, I was dealing with quite the load of stuff. As far as I was concerned, I most definitely had a candida infection. I also had leaky gut syndrome, and I was most certainly hypo-glycemic. I had a host of viruses and bacterial infections in my system, both latent and active, that needed eradication. I was suffering from adrenal fatigue and absolutely had a clogged colon. My white blood cell count was too low, and my body was too acidic. I was lactose intolerant, and I had sensitivities to a laundry list of other foods as well. I had a sluggish lymphatic system, and my hormones were imbalanced. You name it — I was certain I had it.

But of all the new conditions added to my ever-growing list, the Lyme disease diagnosis was the king pin of them all. It was defi-nitely the captain of all the other ailments, with its treatment awarded top priority. In fact, it even superseded my CFS diag-nosis for a while.

When my batch of lab work came back that revealed the positive results for Lyme disease, I latched onto this diagnosis immediately. Lyme disease sounded real, and like something I could put all my energy into and tackle head-on. And most people had actually heard of Lyme disease, which I also thought lent my condition some of the legitimacy I craved. There was a sort of permission I was looking for from others when it came to my illness. I felt really guilty for being off work for so long and for being so unreliable to my colleagues, and I didn't think that CFS sounded serious enough to justify my being out of commission for so long. Lyme disease, on the other hand, was still hard to treat and mysterious, but it wasn't insane. To me, my Lyme disease diagnosis meant that everyone would finally know that I was not crazy, or lazy, and that I had in fact been suffering immensely. It meant that my struggles would be acknowledged, and I could selfishly and without guilt continue to push work, family, and friends to the side while I focused on getting better.

The theory was that some time ago without my noticing I'd been bitten by a Lyme-infected tick. Had the Lyme disease been caught right away, a standard course of antibiotics would've quickly and easily cleared it up. But since I didn't get the telltale bull's eye rash that typically accompanies Lyme disease and signifies to someone that they'd been infected, I wasn't aware that anything had happened. And because the disease had been left to roam freely and untreated in my body for so long, it would now be much more difficult to eradicate, and thus the word *chronic* was added to the diagnosis.

Although the chronic version of this disease appeared to be a much tougher beast to battle, there were definitely documented cases of people getting past this. The more I learned about Lyme, the more hopeful I got. Although I'd always been quite disciplined in my healing plan, this latest news gave me the hope and the buy-in to really, truly buckle down. Every bite of food that went into my mouth was now organic; every single product used in my home was natural and toxin-free. Once I knew with absolute certainty that recovery was possible, no cheat seemed worth the potential cost.

That chronic Lyme disease diagnosis served as a lifeline for me when I most desperately needed one. It was my True North, providing the foremost direction toward which to steer all my healing efforts. I firmly believed that if I cured the Lyme disease, then everything else in my body would go back to normal, and I would be healthy and happy once again.

Dr. M. quickly got to work adjusting my healing plan to tackle this new development. Mostly it was business as usual. The biggest change was the couple months' worth of strong antibiotics that were added to my regimen, which left me weak and nauseated to the point of vomiting some days. But the intensity of it all only served to further my faith that this was healing me, and I had absolutely no problem suffering in service of being cured.

And I took it as a sign that Dr. M. was a pioneer in chronic Lyme disease treatment. He'd actually just returned from an overseas Lyme disease conference just prior to diagnosing me, leaving me certain he was on top of all the latest information and treatments. His casual reference to the Lyme disease books stacked on his bedside table was not lost on me either. I kept wondering, *What are the odds? How did I manage to get an expert for such a rare condition dropped into my lap just when I needed him?*

And yet — no matter how valiantly and faithfully I battled my Lyme diagnosis, I just didn't get any better. Aside from making me even sicker, the endless weeks of antibiotics seemed to accomplish nothing, and eventually my doctor took me off them, and my CFS diagnosis once again prevailed as the main culprit.

Looking back, I can't help but be curious about which came first — the doctor, or the Lyme disease diagnosis. It seems very possible that because his world at the time was so immersed in it, a well-intentioned Dr. M. could potentially have been "seeing" more cases of chronic Lyme disease than actually existed.

And the more I read on chronic Lyme disease, the more I came to realize that this diagnosis was more than a little controversial in the medical community, with not all doctors recognizing it as a legitimate disease. Apparently the testing was unreliable, and scientific recognition of the disease aside, my family's medical history should have raised some red flags for me. Was this three generations of Lyme disease we were seeing in my family? Because no matter how bad Lyme was, the one thing it was not was hereditary.

Since I'm not a doctor or a scientist of any kind, I can't speak to the legitimacy of chronic Lyme disease as a whole. Although it seems likely that some people do legitimately have this disease, I'm not sure I ever actually did. It's amazing how powerful our minds can be, really. At the time, a diagnosis like this was exactly what I needed to keep going, so my mind found a way to let me believe it. If nothing else, Lyme disease served as a lifeline for me. It distracted me from so much of my hopelessness and kept me motivated to keep plugging along at a time when I really needed to keep plugging along.

In time, the World Wide Web would essentially become my mother's doctor and provide her with the CFS diagnosis she had been looking for all along. Trapped at home and glued to her fancy new HP Notebook, it didn't take long for her to find that label for which she'd been desperately searching. A diagnosis of CFS didn't yet come with a detailed prognosis or any hint at a treatment plan, but nevertheless, she was ecstatic to find it. With a name came the starting place for moving forward on what she hoped would be her own healing journey.

My mother marched into her doctor's office with detailed printouts about this newly discovered condition. "I think you are probably right," her physician said after briefly reviewing the papers. "You have chronic fatigue syndrome."

Her doctor seemed happy and relieved to finally have a diagnosis, though not because he thought that they would now have a jumping-off point for treatment. My mother's distinct impression was that her doctor believed that now that she finally had a diagnosis she would just leave him alone. It didn't matter whether or not he actually believed in the CFS diagnosis — he just wanted her gone.

Despite her doctor's reaction, after years without a sensible diagnosis, getting one meant everything to my mother. Now she actually had something to tell people that could explain why she was so sick all the time. Now she actually had something to tell herself as well.

But CFS, at that time, was regrettably not a diagnosis you could share with pride. It was the *Yuppie Flu*, a fashionable form of hypochondria, needy urbanites just seeking attention. A couple years after my mother's self-diagnosis, she would request copies of all her medical files for review. As she flipped through the photocopied pages she discovered that even the GPs and specialists who sounded positive and supportive to her face had made notes in her chart stating that this was all in her head.

One thing was clear: when it came to her illness and her treatment, she was just as much on her own *after* the diagnosis as she was before it. So she stayed glued to her laptop and found online some medications that she thought might help. By this point, her criteria for a *good doctor* was simply someone who would fill whatever prescriptions she asked for without question. To her relief, she found someone who wasn't that interested in the small print on their medical diploma (that part that said *do no harm*). She also managed to wrangle some specialists on the side that would supplement her medicine cabinet with even more prescription medications. Although she had no friends left by this point in time, she definitely made friends with her pills, regularly throwing "parties" of "the more the merrier" sort.

Before long she had a rotating arsenal of pills. There were those she took to help her sleep at night and an equal but opposite batch that helped her wake up in the morning. She took muscle relaxers to help her stiff joints, some pretty hardcore opiates to help her pain, and even threw in a few antipsychotics for good measure. She rotated through a regular catalog of antidepressants and anti-anxiety meds and anything else with even a 1 percent chance of helping her condition improve. The doctors she saw didn't seem to compare notes, and no one seemed aware of her total pill count. She didn't care much about harmful side-effects, and she had no discernible limit.

She would try anything. She was that desperate.

With Lyme disease in my rearview mirror, I plowed ahead in search of new solutions for my health problems. Dr. M. remained my healing guru, but that didn't keep me from seeking out other practitioners and supplementary sages that might be able to also help guide me back to vibrant health.

Although I still generally embraced Western medicine, my love affair with the holistic healing community remained strong and was definitely my focus at that time. I saw colon hydrother-apists and massage therapists and physiotherapists — if there was a therapist for it, I definitely checked it out. I got acupuncture, and I figured out what my dosha was (*Vata* all the way, baby!). A homeopathic doctor sent me off with a bag full of glass bottles filled with what appeared to be water but that, apparently, contained the *essences* of various substances with the ability to cure me.

Maybe it was just modern life that was the culprit. I got tested for allergies and food intolerances and even had my house professionally inspected for mold. I found a dentist who specialized in leaky fillings to ensure I didn't have any hidden mercury leaching into my bloodstream.

One very kind older man I saw worked regularly to clear up my clogged energy meridians. Each visit, as I laid on a table in his office, his hands hovered above my body while he attempted to energetically remove whatever needed removing so that my body could heal. Beads of sweat ran down his face during the process, and after each session, when all was said and done, despite having never touched me, he'd collapse in his office chair panting as if he'd just run a marathon.

One afternoon I also gave something called Family Constellation Therapy a try. Sitting on the constellation thera-pist's living room floor along with half a dozen or so other participants, I closed my eyes and waited curiously for the process to begin. Before I knew it, dead people with tons to say were apparently all around me. And not just any dead people, these were my ancestors, here to join in on today's discussion and talk about fixing my health. Although I could not see or hear any of these dead relatives, others in the room claimed they could and reported back to me everything they heard and saw.

These dead folks apparently talked up a storm, revealing all sorts of family secrets to the group. It was drama galore, with no shortage of rapes and murders divulged. It appeared that unbeknownst to me I had quite the juicy family history, and until these scandalous issues were resolved amongst the deceased, I was told that my body would not be able to heal.

After some time and despite my not being able to actually see any of them, I was assured by the group facilitator that my family members had made amends, shed some tears of joy, and provided me with their support and permission to heal.

Despite this all seeming more than a little wonky to me, I somehow left the session feeling surprisingly uplifted. No matter how unconventional, there's just something about a room full of people that seem invested in your well-being that feels good, regardless of how bizarre the circumstances.

In a more conventional approach to wellness, I also started seeing a psychologist named Priya. She was such a pillar of strength for me and such a hugely supportive person that, should I ever have a child, I would seriously consider naming it after her. No joke — she was that good.

I liked Priya from Day One. Her cleverness and insightfulness kept me on my toes, and I loved that she didn't accept any of my crap. While I was in her office I had to own my life and my choices and focus on fixing only the things that I could control. There would be no blaming others for my problems or issues. Not on her watch. My husband is annoying me? I need to fix me, not him. A friend keeps judging me? The friend is a non-issue. Change myself.

Priya also believed me when I told her I was sick, and as I think I've mentioned only a thousand times already, people believing that my struggles were real was a bit of a hang-up for me at the time. It's hard being told that you are making up the manacles that you can feel around your wrists all the time. She told me stories about her curling her hair in the mornings while thinking how hard it would be to struggle, like me, with even simple tasks like this. And at a time when I still, for whatever reason, suspected that many people thought I was exaggerating my illness, her faith in my struggles meant a lot.

On top of the multitude of practitioners and healers I was seeing, the "basic" at home daily healing regimen that Dr. M. prescribed had also become its own Everest to climb. Despite my rock-bottom energy levels requiring me to spend the majority of my time lying down and resting, I somehow managed to find a way to power through a considerable list of healing activities most days.

First thing in the morning, I would reacquaint myself with that most miraculous of creatures living inside of me: my tongue. Maneuvering it in every possible way, I would get my tongue scraping into action and remove the furry coating of moss that had appeared on it overnight, putting my gag reflex to the test. Of all the various hoops I jumped through at this time, I still to this day perform my morning routine with my tongue. We are best friends, my tongue and I, and while scraping it clean had nothing to do with my eventual recovery, starting the day without my tongue feeling like a Chia Pet seems like a good strategy in general.

I'd then head downstairs to the kitchen to retrieve my container of liquid B12 from the fridge, and with a newly filled syringe I'd reluctantly stab myself in the thigh. Then with some freshly squeezed lemon water and two dozen supplements in hand, I'd plant myself down at the kitchen table and soak up as many healing rays from my light therapy box as I could while popping my pills. During the warmer months I'd go outside onto my backyard deck and into the actual sun for this, but during the long, dreary Canadian winters, this mechanical contraption feebly trying to mimic natural sunlight had to do. As the fake sunlight soaked in, I'd swallow those supplements meant to be taken on an empty stomach and read through my daily list of positive affirmations in an attempt to lift my spirits and keep my motivation to heal in tip-top shape.

Having embraced the fact that I was *perfectly imperfect* and trying hard *not to let the past dictate my future*, I'd head over to my mini trampoline and make like a two-year-old performing some light rebounding exercises. I'd follow these up by executing a couple stretches assigned to me by my energy healer — having forgotten their actual names, I'd refer to them simply as *Rotisserie Chicken* and *Try to Lick Your Elbow*. And then, just before taking my alternating hot and cold shower, I'd get my special soft-bristle brush out from the closet and, as if I were my own pet horse, brush myself from head to toe. Try it sometime, and embrace the My Little Pony inside you too.

Come time for breakfast, when I was up for it, I'd cut a handful of spears from my tray of wheatgrass perched in the kitchen window and liquify them in my fancy juicer. I followed this with a fresh glass of low-glycemic green vegetable juice and then chased that with a tablespoon of coconut oil as well. (If this book doesn't work out I have a hell of a future as a juice-bar barista.) Then, in an effort to ensure I was not taxing my digestive system unnecessarily, as I ate my breakfast I'd count how many times I chewed each mouthful of organic goodness before swallowing. What *kind* of organic I could never settle on: I started out eating vegetarian, then switched to vegan, then went whole hog (so to speak) and embraced raw vegan before eventually returning to my organic omnivorous ways. I'd also swallow another couple dozen supplements that were meant to be taken with food. As the day went on, I'd continue to periodically take handfuls of supplements until my carefully portioned out 104 pills for the day were gone.

I should point out that by this time I'd replaced all my "toxic" plastic food containers with glass ones and my poisonous Teflon cookware with expensive ceramic versions. My newly installed home water-purification system worked overtime to leech out all the biohazards lurking in my unthinkably undrinkable tap water. And I was forever on the verge of getting this particular air ionizer "as seen on TV." I wanted those ions and could just taste the pure air, but I never managed to stay awake long enough to catch the infomercial on the air.

At some point in the day I'd enjoy some episodes of one of my favorite comedy TV series and put in my best effort to receive some of the remarkable healing benefits of laughter that I'd read so much about. Most days a glimpse at the daily activities of my very own life should have been enough to get me roaring, but finding the humor in my own situation was not yet something that I'd mastered. And despite the ridiculous sight of some of these activities, I didn't yet know which ones I should be laughing at, because some items in my daily regimen were actually pulling their weight and slowly getting me some small results. I didn't yet have the faintest idea which ones, but hidden in the rough were definitely some gems.

Occasionally I'd also take the "plunge" and conduct my own home enemas, using a combination of warm water, coffee dregs, and whatever other liquid my most recent cleanse book had advocated. Somewhere in the day I'd consume small portions of bee pollen and bentonite clay for their "remarkable" cleansing and healing properties, and I'd down a smoothie containing scoops of various "superfood" powders in different spectral shades of green. My daily checklist also included resting on my couch counting each slow, deep breath in an effort to ensure that my body was fully oxygenated and swishing coconut oil around in my mouth in an attempt to draw out harmful germs lodged in my teeth and gums. (One thing I can say is that with this, combined with the tongue scraping, my breath had never been fresher.)

Before heading to bed, on the days I could manage it, I'd sweat it out for a bit in my infrared sauna in my basement. And because I'd been told that the infrared waves in the sauna I'd purchased might not be covering enough of the light spectrum (or something to that extent), I quickly went out in search of an additional heat lamp to install that could provide those missing rays. It turned out that the only bulb I could find that covered this extra wavelength requirement was sold exclusively to chicken farmers. And so there I would sit in the evenings before bed under my new chicken lamp as if waiting for my chicks to hatch. (Neither my egg production nor my health saw a discernible uptick.)

Once I finally made it to bed, with my headlamp firmly strapped in place on my forehead, I'd use its light to journal about my potential unconscious motivations for being sick and explore some of the many other important mental aspects of healing. And as I went over my day with a fine-toothed comb, I'd also pull out what small improvements I was seeing in my health and add them to my steadily growing gratitude journal. The headlamp was necessary of course for limiting my exposure to electromagnetic energy. My bedroom electrical outlets always went unused, with no electronics of any sort permitted in the sacred space where I slept (battery-operated lights strapped to my skull having not yet explicitly been outlawed by any of my healing books).

With my journaling complete and my headlamp stored

back inside my bedside table, I'd close my eyes and visualize an imaginary battle in my body of little armies of *good guys* and *bad guys*, one in which the *good guys* obviously always won and left my body in a radiant state of health. As far as I know, this imaginary battle never got me any closer to overcoming CFS during my waking hours, but I do know that I was not ever — ⸰not even once — sick in my dreams.

It was a small victory, but I happily took it.

―――――――

When it came to getting better, nothing was too crazy or too outlandish for me to try. Invisible potions, consulting the dead, "hydro"-anything — bring it on. I made myself my very own CFS lab rat and experimented with it all. And no matter how much I put into my body, I worked twice as hard to make sure it left. Like any good holistic health patient, I did a ton of cleanses.

It seems like any alternative health book worth its salt must include a vital cleanse of some sort, and whatever I read about, I always tried. I did liver cleanses where I'd chug concoctions of olive oil and laxatives and cleanses where I only ate blended foods. I did elimination diet cleanses to try and find the seemingly innocent culprits that might be hiding in my food and conspiring to ruin my health. I did cleanses where I consumed nothing but lemon water with cayenne pepper and maple syrup (anyone else remember the so-called "Master Cleanse"?!), as well as an endless array of juice cleanses lasting anywhere from one day to one week in duration. I definitely wasn't alone or in any way special in doing some of these. With cleanses being all the rage at that time, in Canada, much of the population at large got swept up right along with me with a couple of these.

But the cleanse of all cleanses, the one that all other cleanses aspired to be when they grew up, was a four-week ten-thousand-dollar body purification marathon I did in the Sonoran desert.

Shortly after watching a documentary promoting the apparent healing powers of a raw food diet, I found myself on a plane headed to the Arizona rejuvenation center where it had been filmed. With my slowly increasing energy levels, I tentatively embarked on this cross-country excursion hoping that my body would hold up long enough to survive this little experiment. When I arrived at this health retreat of sorts, that was located just a fifteen-minute drive from the Mexican border and immersed in fields of cactuses and free-roaming pig-like animals known as javelinas, I wasn't quite sure what I'd gotten myself into.

I've never been to a hippie commune before, but in my mind, this rejuvenation center was exactly what I imagined one would look like. Small meditation temples, fresh vegetable greenhouses, and platforms meant for naked sunbathing peppered the serene grounds of this place. Barefoot and hemp-clad individuals with names like Sunflower and Koala moseyed about, offering up, with their hands pressed flat together as if in prayer, gentle smiles and soft utterances of *namaste* as they passed by.

For those guests at this center whose cleansing programs included the consumption of solid food, a raw vegan buffet was prepared three times a day for meals, with much of the food made to resemble more conventional dishes such as sushi, pizza, and bread. For those guests, such as myself, who were partaking in a mostly liquid-based diet, a large fridge was stocked each morning with mason jars filled with freshly made low-glycemic green vegetable juice.

Energy levels permitting, my mornings at this place began

each day at 5:00 a.m., when wrapped in a thick blanket I'd sleepily stumble out into the chilly pre-dawn air and make my way to sunrise meditation. In a quaint stone meditation temple that was no more than ten square meters (about 100 square feet) in size, a few guests and the meditation leader would gather and begin the group meditation. In this tiny building that was situated on top of what was said to be a positive energy-emitting vortex, we silently welcomed the day, honoring the sun as a conscious entity modeling for us the giving of light and warmth to others.

Granted, many guests chose to skip this morning meditation in favor of a couple more hours of sleep. But health permitting, this over-achiever right here did every single thing that this center had to offer. I was forking over a lot of cash for my stay, and I absolutely wanted to get my money's worth. And who was to say which item on my itinerary might or might not be the activity with the power to heal me? I certainly wasn't going to chance it by skipping anything for a couple more lousy hours of sleep. I felt that during this last year or two I had banked enough sleep to last me a lifetime.

For the bulk of my twenty-eight days spent at this healing center, I consumed nothing but green juice. To help ease me into and out of the juicing program, I was given a couple days at the start and end of my stay where I could eat the food from the raw vegan buffet. While those few days spent grazing the buffet of salads and faux sushi were pleasing and enjoyable, the three straight weeks of consuming absolutely nothing but small portions of watered-down celery and spinach juice were punishing. Breakfast: here's your tiny glass of water juice. Lunch: same. Dinner? How would you like fifty more calories of liquid to tide you over until morning? And to top it off, being in such a serene and slow-paced environment meant that I had very little to distract me from the debilitating weakness, shortness of breath, and gnawing hunger pangs from the lack of food.

It was a tough program, but no one was forcing it on me. When I signed up to come I specifically selected this plan from the menu of available options. I chose what looked like the most extreme option on the list because if I was going to come all this way and spend all this money, I might as well go all-in and try to get the most out of it that I could.

Because I often felt quite sick and weak during this juice cleanse I unfortunately had to spend much of my time in bed, but over the 4 weeks I somehow still managed to take part in quite a few of the activities the center had to offer. After I finished my sunrise meditation and green juice breakfast, I might head to a class on conscious writing or raw food preparation. Then, after a nap and if I felt up to it, I'd take part in a qigong or kundalini yoga class. I could never finish them, but I did what I could. After some more rest, I might head for a lymphatic drainage massage where the therapist would on occasion pause to communicate with the bees outside because she was sure that their buzzing contained some important messages meant just for her.

On the days I could muster the motivation and the courage, in the shared bathrooms with faulty locks on the doors I'd nervously complete the self-conducted enemas that this facility insisted were absolutely essential for good health. And there were, of course, weekly colonics to conduct as well. Throughout the day I'd take breaks to periodically measure the pH levels of my urine and saliva, and no matter how much I cleansed I always failed to meet the target levels set by the rejuvenation center, with both my pee and my spit remaining stubbornly acidic. I also took part in hydrotherapy sessions where I'd alternate between taking a cold shower and sitting in what looked and felt like a giant hot egg.

When all the cleansing for the day was done, sometimes I'd pop into the Dharma Room where, after having washed one another's hands and feet, guests would feed each other freshly made juice and raw bread (for those who were eating solid food) in a spiritual community-building exploration of one another. These typically included seemingly endless discussions about the higher consciousness perceptions of our Third Eye (and the impending 2012 Mayan calendar disaster as well).

Most evenings were quite relaxed, with guests often congregating after dinner around the communal juicer for some shots of wheatgrass. Occasionally, before heading to bed, I'd take part in one of the nightly fire ceremonies on the grounds, taking in the rhythmic sounds and sights of the guitars, drums, chanting, singing, and swaying, with people sometimes even howling at the moon.

One night I even took part in my first ever sweat lodge ceremony with a small group inside a dark dome-shaped hut, with glowing red-hot rocks radiating from the center, where I sat in a state of intense distress and wondered if I would survive the suffocating heat. The glowing rocks gave off so much heat that I seriously worried I might pass out, so although this was meant to be a peaceful ceremony for prayer, purification, and healing, for me, it was unfortunately not much more than an exercise in dealing with panic.

Just before each day was about to wrap up, I'd find myself back in that same quaint stone temple in which I'd started the day, finishing things off with one last bit of meditation. Since there was meditation included in virtually every activity we did, it wasn't unusual for me to rack up three or more hours of meditation each day.

The center radically redefined priorities and threw out conventional beliefs about how to live a happy and healthy life. The people at this healing center made their own simpler, quieter rules that were more in tune with nature, and I suspect that many people, guests and staff alike, came here for just that reason.

And regardless of what clothes and accessories the guests at this place arrived with, before long, we all started to resemble one another. It only took a few days for us to stop using hair products and makeup, and after a visit to the clothing section of the gift shop, we quickly all fell in line with the free-spirited bohemian fashions of the staff at this center. We rapidly became a community of sorts, identifiable by our unofficial uniforms and unified by a collective desire to learn about a healthier and more natural way of living.

Throughout my stay, different guests shared with me some of their beliefs about the benefits of eating only uncooked food. Many appeared to believe that eating a raw food diet allowed your body to function in an almost superhuman capacity, impervious to any number of afflictions.

One afternoon, someone explained to me that the sunscreen that I was smearing all over my body was unnecessary because people who eat raw food don't get sunburns. And it was of course also just plain crazy to try and put any sort of barrier between myself and something as natural as the sun. Sunglasses were also shunned because we were always, at all times, to let the healing powers of the sun in. And as much as possible, we should also ditch our shoes and walk around barefoot so that we could absorb the healing powers of the earth. On this diet, our bodies were said to function so optimally that childbirth wasn't even painful. One afternoon a guest at this center even ate some pine needles he'd collected because, as far as he was concerned, all things that nature provided were good for us.

And it apparently wasn't just humans who'd messed up the proper order of things by moving to a cooked, omnivorous diet. One talk I attended that was put on by the medical doctor who ran this facility discussed the shift in consciousness that was in the works — one in which all species on our planet were becoming more harmonious. This physician explained that animals would soon stop eating one another and that a planet of vegans, across all species, was on the horizon and would be a reality very soon.

Despite my not quite buying into everything I heard, this healing center nevertheless introduced a whole new world to me and got me thinking about an entirely different approach to living. The admittedly quirky people at this rejuvenation center felt so open, so natural, and so beautifully and blissfully raw. Magical things seemed to happen at this healing hippie commune of sorts, with bonds forming between people so much more quickly and easily than I had ever experienced before. The difficult life circumstances that'd brought many of the guests there showed me that when it comes to building relationships, facing hardship often enables people to strip away the fluff and zero-in on what's important. I quickly noticed that small talk is a privilege of the healthy and happy, whereas real talk is a blessing bestowed on the troubled.

This raw food center also attracted interesting guests from all over the world. One impossibly tall and stunning British woman whose wardrobe could only be described as *vampire chic* had come to this place to do research for the raw food restaurant she was opening in London. Over lunch one day I sat starstruck as I casually chatted up another guest who was the maker of a vegan diet documentary I'd recently seen. Being knee-deep in the holistic health world at the time, this man was nothing short of a celebrity to me, and I was beyond stoked to have the opportunity to talk with him. I also made friends with a wild and fascinating woman with cancer who, in an attempt to heal herself, had flown to this Arizona center all the way from Australia.

I was connecting with such a diverse range of wonderful people and having life-changing experiences at this place almost each and every day. At the end of just my first week at this center, I pronounced it to be one of the best weeks of my life. And by the end of my stay, I was still incredibly grateful for the experience and so happy that I'd decided to come. I'd arrived feeling completely stressed out and at my wit's end, and when I left I felt so much more at peace. I left feeling hopeful and full of so much love, gratitude, and joy. This place served as a personal growth bootcamp for me and provided a much-needed dose of spiritual nutrition.

This center unfortunately didn't "cure" me, but I'd learned so much and met so many great people that I definitely had zero regrets. When I left the rejuvenation center, despite still being sick, my body somehow felt like a shiny brand-new car, fresh off the lot, and because of this I thought more carefully about what I put into it and how I treated it. Although I hadn't yet reached my goal of overcoming CFS, I felt as if generally in life I was getting closer to eventually understanding how this would be possible and was more on the right track.

By that point in time, in the year and a half that'd passed since I'd first gotten sick, I'd managed to recover by about 50 percent. I wasn't really sure at that point what was helping me and what wasn't, so as much as I could, I kept doing it all. It wasn't the best way to live, but I was getting by, and I didn't know what else to do; I was definitely running out of things to try.

Those intense early days of discovery ended up being invaluable for me. I'd needed that time to explore and learn about health and my body so that I could move forward. The retreat marked a milestone for me: after it, for the first time, I thought that some aspects of CFS might have moved into my rearview mirror and that regular oil changes and tune-ups might keep the worst of it at bay.

Little did I know that I'd soon have to completely rebuild the jalopy that was my life from scratch.

4

LETTING GO

You might wonder what for me was the hardest part of confronting CFS. The food regimen was serious business, and the various cleanses were demanding in the extreme. Burning a hole in my bank account was no joke, and of course the soul-crushing fatigue I felt in my bones sometimes felt like a minute-by-minute battle. But the emotional toll CFS would take on me was truly devastating. And in my heart of hearts, I knew this was going to be the case, because of what had happened to my mom.

Her first hard years with CFS turned into decades, and my mother's condition continued to steadily deteriorate, with a seemingly endless trail of research, doctors, medications, therapies, and various healing potions bringing her no relief. No matter what she tried, my mother's health never saw an uptick or even a plateau. As the disease progressed and the years marched onward, she was largely house-ridden, often bedridden, and always miserable. When her CFS was at its worst, my mother was only able to leave the house in a wheelchair. Yet despite her lengthy battle with CFS, she never really accepted this illness as a part of her life. Whatever energy she could muster she used to rage against this disease.

As selfish as this sounds, almost worse still was how her sickness wore on the rest of us. Living with CFS in our home made my father and I often feel like we were trapped in some sort of pressure cooker.

"It might be best to not even mention to Mom that we went out for lunch today," I suggested hesitantly to my dad one Sunday afternoon as he and I made our way to our cars in the Applebee's parking lot. The look of unease on his face told me that he was, without question, as intimidated as I by the thought of having that conversation with her.

"Let's just say we were each out running errands. No need to upset her," we quickly agreed.

Family joy — when experienced in my mother's absence — was forbidden. It certainly hadn't always been that way, but as time marched on it became clear that this new rule was true. It was a tough one to abide by, and over the years my father and I got worse and worse at keeping up our end of this dictated bargain.

One Saturday morning, with a note left hesitantly on the kitchen counter serving as the first and only notice explaining our whereabouts, like rebellious teenagers my father and I piled into the car and made our way to a wedding celebration a couple hours' drive outside the city.

Due to her turned-around sleeping schedule, it was late in the afternoon and the wedding was well underway by the time my mother found her way to our note in the kitchen, and I got my first dreaded phone call from her.

"How could you do this!" she screamed through her tears

into the phone. "Do you have any idea what it feels like to not be able to be a part of something like this?"

As per usual, as a family we'd absolutely discussed the possibility of attending this wedding together. There was no way, my mother assured us, that she could ever dream of making it. It was too far, she'd have to get up too early, and her energy levels would never be enough to get her through the whole day. So without the words ever needing to be said, it was settled. None of us were going.

If a trip to Applebee's without my mother was frowned upon, then a road trip to take part in a large-scale family bash was on par with committing murder. This is in large part why we typically missed most weddings. In fact, until that Saturday we missed *all* weddings. But for whatever reason, come that Saturday my dad and I felt we just didn't want to miss one more. I'd expected a reaction from her, to be sure. That didn't surprise me. But what *did* surprise me was the ferocity with which she came at me on that summer day. Things that for so long went assumed but unsaid — regardless of how irrational they sounded when said out loud — were now outright stated.

"Until *I* am able to attend things like this, *none* of us go," my mother shrieked into the phone with a fierceness that would petrify anyone. "It isn't fair for me to be the only one to have to miss out on things!"

Each time I managed to get off the phone it wouldn't take long before the phone would be ringing once again, and these persistent juvenile rants to ensure that without her I, in fact, did *not* enjoy any family time at this wedding were definitely a success. With my barely controlled sobs and tears continually streaming down my face, I became the unruly wedding guest that my father sat next to sullenly and everyone else doggedly avoided. With each subsequent phone call my mother's sharp words hit their target with more and more precision, tapping into my already-crippling guilt over her pervasive suffering in the face of my ability to live.

For years, life with my mother had meant bearing witness to her heart-wrenching suffering and sadness and grief. But as time wore on, life was more often than not spent navigating a minefield of her acute depression and jealousy and rage. Most of the time we didn't know what to do or how to keep going. It wasn't just that everything ended up revolving around her illness — it was demanded that it be so. And as the years progressed, as a family we definitely shared more tears of pain than joy.

The only thing scarier for me than her demands and accusations was her silence. Because as debilitating as her physical illness and resulting needs were, my mother's depression was even worse. Hours could pass, sometimes even days, where she'd sit at the kitchen table or lie on the couch in complete stillness and silence with a haunting and lifeless look in her eyes. If she was feeling anything like I was feeling on my worst days, in those moments she knew there wasn't a hole small enough for her to crawl into that could shut out the pain brought from just being alive. There was nothing that could console her or convince her that her days still had meaning, or that her life at all resembled anything that she even deigned to live. With each passing day she slowly gave up hope of recovery.

As early on as my adolescence (and long before the clandestine Applebee's trips) the holidays became especially hard because my mother could no longer even mask the deep pain she was in with the spirit of whatever was being celebrated. I used to especially love Christmas and Halloween, but CFS had sucked all the joy out of these holidays. The toddlers stuffed into furry bear costumes and older kids trying to get the idea of their costumes across despite their outfits being squeezed over their bulky winter clothing used to be some of our family's favorite things to witness. As the children yelled repeatedly in unison, *Trick or treat!* while standing next to the pumpkin on our front step that my father had nervously watched me carve, we'd dole out treats and smiles and happiness. But after a while the noise and commotion of all of this had become too much for my mother to bear, so Halloween turned into nights spent with the lights off while we sat in silence and pretended not to be home.

Christmastime was sacred to my mother, so no matter how bad she felt she did what she could to keep some traditions going for this holiday. By the time Christmas had rolled around in 2007 my family had settled into a predictable routine. It began much like all the rest as my husband and I joined my mother and father at my childhood home for dinner. We ate the turkey and stuffing that Dad had lovingly put together (my mother far past being able to prepare meals by this point, much less eat with anything approaching gusto) and enjoyed some nice wine. As the carols that I'd loved since childhood played softly in the background, we made our way through our mountain of gifts under the Christmas tree.

At the end of the night, with both our bellies and hands full, my husband and I stood at the front door of my parents' home and prepared to head out into the cold and make our way home. As we put on our boots, we said goodnight, and I unknowingly hugged my mother goodbye for the last time. After we left, and without telling anyone of her plans, she swallowed a pile of prescription medications that she had been stockpiling. She went to bed and never woke up again.

My own battle with CFS would start just a year later, and there is no doubt that my mother's death haunted my every step. The shadow of her long decline and depression was a shadow cast over everything. Despite witnessing her years of despair and hopelessness, her death still shocked me. And despite the strain and upheaval of having her in my life, her death still devastated me. The person who, regardless of how sick she was, had made sure I had my favorite homemade chocolate cake for every single birthday, the person who'd caressed my head and cared for me each and every time I was sick, and the person who'd poured out affection and loved and supported me with that specific kind of ferocity that only a mother can muster — that person was gone. And although that person had been gone for years, there was always a part of me that held out hope that she would get better and return to her old self. Although I didn't yet appreciate the impact that such intense grief had on my body, the sadness and pain that followed her passing most certainly served as one of the final blows for my own health.

It's quite one thing to grieve for your mother; it's quite another to discover that you have the disease that eventually killed her. Instead of my CFS diagnosis being the beacon of light that it initially was for my mother, for me it carried the jolt of a death sentence. Every single memory I had of my mother was fused with something ugly highlighting the devastation of CFS. A clearer picture of what was to come could not possibly have been painted. I knew the sickening road that was ahead, and I absolutely wanted no part of it.

Just as I should have seen my illness coming given my family history, I should have seen how my marriage would be affected by CFS given our history as a couple. But when your only tool for dealing with the tough stuff is denial, you are primed for surprises.

Those surprises started to arrive as I entered my thirties — not as right hooks to the chin, but as lightning-quick body blows that made me catch my breath but think that I could wade back in and avoid more punishment (while getting in some punches myself). Things like my husband telling me one random after- noon that he and the boys tried to flip a car last night when coming home from a bar, and listening to the pride ringing in his voice as he boasted, "I wanted to see if I was strong enough to do it."

"But that's *someone's car!*" I responded, with the horror I felt certainly radiating from my face. "What if someone did that to *your* car? How would *you* feel?" But my entreaties made no dent in his armor — he was a boy and resolutely determined to stay that way (particularly with a load on).

In those moments there was clarity — small breaks in my armor of denial where I saw as clear as day a giant red flag waving brightly above his head. Admittedly, if he'd said those same words to me when we'd first started dating, I probably would have laughed and reached for another tequila shot myself. But we were now both firmly in our thirties, and I'd hoped we'd grown up a bit since those days. I'd felt that that one statement spoke volumes about what he wanted his life to look like and how different that was from what I now envi- sioned for mine.

———

I can't blame him for perhaps thinking that it was me that had changed from when we first met. And I had. When we'd first connected it all felt very much like I was a character on *Friends*, as if I were his Rachel and he my Ross. But instead of at a coffee shop, we found ourselves at a small pub where our bartending jobs had us working together — mixing drinks and sneaking shots of tequila — all while denying our mutual attraction for the better part of every week. Each night when we rung last call and the customers finally went home, we'd help ourselves to (read: steal) as much draft beer as we could manage while sharing stories and laughs until the wee hours of the morning.

Everyone else who worked at that pub knew and openly stated that he and I were after each other — everyone except for us. We'd work to creatively find as many platonic opportunities to spend time with each other as we could, but for months it never went past that — until a group trip to the Mayan Riviera with friends finally gave us both the opportunity we'd been looking for. It took a new time zone, sand between the toes, and of course more tequila to experience that magical sensation of freedom you feel in the presence of someone else whose only focus is you. The spell of denial and fear of rejection that we'd been trapped in for so long was broken.

After only a few weeks together as a couple we were so tight that people assumed we'd been that way for years. Despite still living with our parents and never knowing (or asking) how they felt about this arrangement, we rarely spent a night apart. We were inseparable, and if our parents ever wanted to see us then they were going to have to accept that we were a package deal — and they had better get over any old-fashioned ideas about the appropriateness of premarital sleepovers. I needed to wear a sweatshirt of his doused in his intoxicating cologne just to get through the rare times we were apart. His absence felt like it physically hurt. I was infatuated. I was in love.

After we'd finally scraped together enough cash to move out of our respective childhood homes, and each spent a healthy stint learning about life with roommates and fumbling with independence in our bachelor and bachelorette pads, we eventually settled into that first modest townhouse of ours together (the one with which I'd pushed and persevered unpacking like a madman so that we could move into it in a single day). Soon after, we set off on our second tropical vacation together. Once again harvesting the confidence and freedom that came with yet another new time zone, on a magazine-worthy white-sand Cuban beach, he clumsily retrieved a ring box from his pocket and squeaked out some words about wanting to marry me. The ring — a thin band with some tiny diamond flecks embedded — was quite humble, and he quickly clarified that it was just a stand-in to use until we could get back home and go pick out the ring of my dreams. I told him that whatever ring he was giving me right then on that beach with his proposal was the only ring I would ever want. I wanted *him*. I was over the moon to be marrying him, and his beautiful love was all I could ever dream of wanting in life.

Our dating life was intimately wound up with alcohol, but I don't want to give the impression that somehow it was fueled by alcohol. (Ok, initially it probably was. Like I said, denial is a powerful force.) Historically, if either one of us was ever going to be accused of pushing the limits with the drinks, anyone you asked would definitely tell you it would be me. Although it would be many years before I would come close to mastering the delicate skill of moderation, CFS instantly taught me abstinence. And since my husband always seemed to have a *take it or leave it* attitude toward booze, once I got sick and pulled the plug on alcohol it ceased to exist in our home.

Until one day when I noticed its abrupt reemergence. I caught myself asking, "Hey, how come you're having a drink every day when you get home from work all of a sudden?" He'd hesitated and just looked at me, and I'd plunged on. The booze itself didn't bother me; it was this sudden out-of-the-blue change of behavior with alcohol after all these years. "You seem kind of quiet and tense much of the time. Everything ok?" Something was clearly going on with him, but "Yep, everything's fine," was all I ever got in response. I could have pushed for more information, but I was deluged with information dealing with my CFS diagnosis and, as shown above, had made myself way too busy to really devote the attention to my marriage it needed.

But I realize now that in those moments I was also recognizing that we were not at all on track with the plan that *I'd* had for our lives — that something was going on with me, not him. By this point we were to be sophisticated and worldly and in a perpetual state of growth. And we were — at all times — to follow *my* plan for how our lives would go. We were to always grow together, in the exact same direction (my direction) and at the exact same speed (my speed). *What the hell was going on?* Didn't he get the memo?

By now, I'd imagined that with our old-fashioned gender stereotypes long ago tossed out the window, he'd be navigating the kitchen with ease while casually preparing us whatever latest dish he'd seen on his favorite cooking channel. As he braised the roast and julienned the vegetables, we'd expertly utilize the skills we'd learned at our latest effective communication course and sort through any marital issues that currently required our attention. We would sip our kombucha and move on to discuss whether we wanted to next put our efforts into finding an overseas job placement for a couple years, or perhaps instead tack on an additional university degree to our credentials. Then, as we savored our dinner, we'd laugh about that ungraceful fall I'd taken while at our most recent hot yoga class together, before we finally settled in for the night in front of our majestic fireplace to watch a documentary and learn about the most effective ways to prevent further climate change.

———

If I'm being completely honest, he wasn't the only one not communicating. As our years together moved along I'd frequently felt like things with us weren't as they should be, but instead of discussing it with him I'd pour my heart out in my journal in a desperate attempt to make sense of it all. *He never seems to want to spend time with me. Ever. I am his last choice for a companion all the time. I am not Plan B — I am Plan Z. The bottom of the totem pole. I have to literally book his time on the weekend in advance if I want to see him. I have to book time with my own husband! How can someone who claims to love me so much also make me feel so invisible and unwanted?*

It wasn't that I'd needed him to entertain me. Self-motivated and always rotating through hobbies, I had no shortage of things to keep me occupied. By September I'd usually already have a box of expertly handcrafted Christmas cards addressed and ready to go. My home pedicures were always on point and my house always spotless. I could decorate and organize and bake the days away without ever feeling even a blip of boredom. And as you can tell, once CFS reared its ugly head I had plenty of other things to occupy my time.

Loneliness — now that was a different story.

Meanwhile, for him it was days spent on the golf course, hours enthralled by his online poker tournaments, hell — even happily volunteering for weekends spent helping friends move. They were evidently *all* more appealing options than hanging out with his wife. He was a *guy's guy* through and through; I don't think I ever really stood a chance. And a CFS diagnosis doesn't change that but amplifies it. He would go out for a beer with friends, and I would stay home with a coffee enema.

Although this all started long before illness entered the equation, CFS certainly worsened our separation. Although he originally did not have much use for his PlayStation, after my health issues set in these games suddenly kept him locked away in his man cave for hours on end. And double shifts taken at work under the guise of making extra money to cover my medical bills felt more and more like a way to avoid the clinical atmosphere and teary-eyed wife that had taken over our home.

As time went on I eventually started looking down at my little engagement ring with regret while cursing myself for not accepting that offer for a better one. For naively not realizing that in the lonely years that would eventually come I would be crying out for some sort of visible indicator of my importance in this relationship. That that ring and how quickly he accepted that I didn't require from him a better one could be an early sign of how much I was valued as a partner — and as an even more important indicator of how much I valued myself.

Another *tiny* hint years earlier that something was amiss that probably should have grabbed my attention: I'd started fantasizing about him *dying*.

I never set out with the intention of having these thoughts; I'd just randomly catch myself having them. Relaxing in the backyard while soaking up the sun I'd realize I was in the middle of a full-blown fantasy where he'd died in a car accident, and (after an acceptable grieving period of course) I was working my new fast-paced job in some exotic overseas place. Or perhaps I was deep in the embrace of the arms of some dreamy man with an intense desire for me emanating from his piercing eyes every single time he looked at me. Whatever the fantasy, I was always doing something adventurous or falling into the arms of a man who couldn't get enough of me.

I in no way actually wanted my husband dead. He was in all the ways that truly matter a wonderful human being, and the world by far was a better place with him in it. This was apparently just the only scenario in which I could imagine myself able to (guilt-free) live the life that I *actually* wanted to be living. These fantasies of being in a relationship with someone who truly adored and desired me even persisted into the night and made their way into my dreams, and when I'd wake in the morning I'd have to shake the depression that always came with the realization that, sadly, I was still mostly on my own, and none of it had been real.

Back in the real world, for years my husband and I had certainly never looked at each other with even a modicum of that intensity or desire I'd seen in my fantasies and dreams. For too long we'd neglected the fire of both our emotional and physical intimacy and let the sparks die. And we never argued. I could see how that might actually sound like a good thing, but it really just meant that nothing of importance in the relationship was ever being addressed. And with him out of town for work more often than he was home (and with this being the pre-smartphone era), much of our correspondence consisted of swift and superficial email exchanges.

As the years passed and we slowly replaced the partying with other hobbies, we found we had less and less in common. Instead of our pool of mutual friends growing and solidifying over time as it sometimes does with couples, our groups had diverged and formed two disconnected crowds with which we each separately spent our time. We ate dinner on our own, went to the gym on our own, and relaxed on our own. Like two single people living as roommates, we kept completely separate schedules. And what little time we did spend together had become draining, with my focus on all that was wrong with us sucking the life right out of me.

Our bank statements even revealed the glaring separateness in our relationship, with our individual credit card expenditures not even coming close to being on par with what our shared bank account could cover. Even with our growing debt displayed for us each month clearly in black and white, we'd refused to compromise and get on the same page. And not trusting him to do anything at all at our home, I took over everything. And then I complained about having to do it all. I had one excuse after another to delay us having kids, and he had just as many excuses for why we shouldn't get counseling or work on making things better with us. We weren't at all a team, and no one had anyone's back — together, we were rarely happy.

Through the years of distance and silence it's not surprising that some strong and destructive feelings had been brewing under the surface for both of us, accumulating and building up pressure while testing the integrity of our emotional walls. *Why did I get married just to spend so much time alone?* Stuff it down. *Why does she have to control everything I do? And are we ever going to have kids?* Stuff it down. *Why won't he support my doing an overseas internship? Has she turned into her mother? Why is he so old-fashioned?* Stuff. It. All. Down.

Despite often feeling rejected and lonely in my marriage, I rarely talked to my husband about it. I never wanted to rock the boat. Staying quiet in an attempt to keep the peace was definitely my MO. It was both of ours. So when we reached a communication crisis it rocked my world.

It was like I was watching it happen to someone else. I heard a cry: feral, raw, and shattered. But since I was the only person in the room, that guttural sound must have come from me. Somehow I'd rolled off my chair and fallen to the floor, with my body apparently no longer functional enough to remain seated. As I laid sobbing and curled in the fetal position on the carpet of our home office, I tried to absorb the words I'd just read and typed in a fateful email exchange with my husband.

"If we don't make some significant changes soon, I might be reaching my breaking point with us," I'd hesitantly wrote, trying to sound serious enough to finally get his attention but not so serious as to completely close any doors. "If things keep going the way they've been going, then I might be done."

This was the first time either one of us had ever even hinted at the possibility of separation. So I thought I was being tough. I was laying down the law and finally standing up for myself and for what I deserved. I was setting the stage for the hard work and serious changes that were going to have to happen very soon if we were going to stay together. My husband would be a bit stung by my harsh words — but he *needed* to hear them.

I braced myself for his response of shock and hurt, but instead, I was the one who was about to be shocked and hurt.

"I think we were done six months ago," was all I got in reply.

And because I too knew deep down that his words were the truth – with those few simple keystrokes my marriage was over.

The fact that this was all determined through email reveals a lot about our relationship. Although we'd been happy and in love for much of our eleven years together, open face-to-face communication was definitely not one of our strengths. I didn't ever tell him what was bothering me, and he returned the favor. It was practically written into our marriage vows. Saying in that fateful email that our marriage had ended only six months prior was being kind.

In truth, the *serious changes* I'd hoped to elicit in that email were to change him into someone else completely. It turns out, as smart as I thought I was at the time, he was smarter. He didn't want to go to counseling. He didn't want to try to fix us. And as much as that hurt, it was exactly the right decision.

By the time my very first CFS symptom made its appearance, our marriage was already a dead man walking. Sure, with my poor health the gap between us widened, but this illness didn't create any problems that weren't firmly already there. We didn't know it, but for years we'd been building a bomb, and CFS was simply the detonator.

After my illness disintegrated our automated and mindless routines, there wasn't much left, and CFS, with all its destruction, finally blew up something useful. That persistent and pervasive denial that had kept our marriage afloat was completely destroyed, and the moment my health improved just enough to enable us to switch our focus from CFS to us, we were finally able to face in our marriage all that needed to be faced and finally say our goodbyes.

Despite our discontent, losing my marriage — *losing my husband* — devastated me. I loved him immensely. I'd felt certain that we'd grow old together and countless times I'd envisioned in detail what that would be like. His morning hugs and occasional cuddles on the couch before bed were the absolute best part of my world. Those were the moments where I could catch a glimpse of what once was. Even as our relationship broke down and all that was left was a shell of what we used to be, deep inside I held onto how loving and devoted we were in the beginning. I held onto those blissful butterfly feelings of his initial love and infatuation. I kept waiting for them to come back. For him to find his way back to looking and me and loving me in that same way. Life with him was all that I knew. And in spite of often feeling hurt and sad while married to him, that life was still somehow all that I wanted to know. With him gone it felt like one of my limbs had been ripped off, as if a vital and treasured piece of who I was had suddenly disappeared.

I looked around despondently at the four plain walls that made up my new world and very slowly exhaled. In no time at all I'd found myself living back with my father in my childhood home and sleeping in my mother's old room. My mother's relentless sleeping difficulties had meant that my parents had to sleep in separate bedrooms, and after my mother had passed away my father was just never able to move back into that master bedroom. It was, after all, the room that she'd died in, but I tried not to let that bother me. After having just given up my entire dream house, I told myself I was just happy to be getting the biggest room.

My zero-gravity plastic reclining lawn chair — the one I used to lean back and relax in while soaking up the sun on the deck attached to my fabulous home — had now been downgraded to the foot of the bed in my mother's old bedroom-turned-bachelorette pad. And since my unceasing CFS symptoms meant that a recent short-lived attempt at a return to work had failed miserably, me and that chair were now better friends than ever. When I couldn't even manage to get through the initial part-time gradual return-to-work schedule, I'd decided it was time to finally quit outright.

Unemployed, chronically ill, newly divorced, and hanging out in my dad's house in my plastic lawn chair, I had so much time to think. *I've tried absolutely everything to get better. There's nothing left to try! This, right here, is as good as it's ever going to get. I'm never going to be able to be independent or support myself again. I will never be able to exercise or be physically active in any capacity ever again. I will never date again. How could anyone possibly ever want me? This is it. Me and this fucking plastic chair. Till death do us part. This is my life now.*

Whatever positive outlook I'd gained at that Arizona healing center felt long gone. Despite knowing that I was really fortunate to have someplace so loving and supportive to land after my husband and I separated, I still felt really sorry for myself. More than that, I felt defeated. Shattered. Beaten down and hopeless. I had tried everything that every kind of medicine I could find had to offer, and this 50 percent improvement was all that it got me. To someone who's never had CFS, I bet 50 percent sounds like it should be enough. Enough to suck it up and just get on with life. Enough to be grateful for what you have. To just deal with it.

That 50 percent — with no hope of any further improvement — is nothing more than a cruel tease. It's taking a starving person all the way to a buffet and then not letting them eat. *But getting here was half the battle — you should just be happy!*

I needed to get off the treadmill of struggle and pain and tears and frustration and hopelessness. And as cliché as this sounds, I really did need to find myself. Life had been suffocating me for too long, and I needed to find a way to breathe again.

Staring at my online savings account balance, I realized that the only thing I had left going for me was money. Even after paying off our somewhat sizable debts, the profits from the sale of our house meant that my ex-husband and I each walked away from our marriage with a decent amount of cash. The only question was: *How could I turn that money into some happiness? Into a reason for living?*

The silver lining of everything in my life falling apart was that I was suddenly accountable to no one, and there was nothing left to stand in my way. If I wanted to spend every penny of that money on bouncy castles or collectible dolls, I didn't need anyone's permission — I could just do it. And crawling into my plastic chair and getting on my laptop to explore places to go spend that money was the only thing that gave me a reason to continue getting out of bed every morning.

Should I go to Hawaii? Or Costa Rica? No — scratch that — Australia! Oh, wait, it's winter there now. That certainly won't do. But Australia sounds awesome. What warm place can I go hang out in that's close to Australia while I wait for their scorching Aussie summer to arrive? Thailand? Yes. YES! Oh my God definitely Thailand.

My health still mostly sucked, but I was prepared to crawl around the globe on my hands and knees if I had to. So after settling on the Thailand-Australia plan, I opened a new tab on my laptop and took another look at my savings account balance. As far as I could guesstimate, I could manage a six-month budget trip and still have a little left over when all was said and done. I realize that any sensible person with no hope of employment in the foreseeable future would likely have hung on for dear life to every penny that they had, but at this point in time I was feeling anything but sensible. It was time to pull out the stops and time to find a way to start living again. I wanted to break free from my bubble of suffering and immerse myself in adventure and distract myself from the ever-present diagnosis of CFS. I wanted to be someplace where no one knew that I was sick and nothing reminded me of what I'd gone through during those last few years.

And *anything* sounded better than continuing to hang out in my plastic chair in my dead mother's bedroom.

Aside from picking a country to start out in and buying a plane ticket, for once in my life I didn't plan a single thing. With nothing but a backpack and some hope for the future in tow, I boarded my flight to Bangkok.

III

PLANNING MY ESCAPE

5
_____

FALSE STARTS

Standing with my feet immersed in the cool and clear water of Hat Maya Beach, I noticed that I was crying. But something was different about these tears — these weren't the same tears of pain and sadness I'd become so accustomed to shedding in recent years. These tears right here were something new. Something forgotten and foreign. These tears were tears of *joy*.

Even though I was still every bit as sick as I'd been in Canada, being all alone on the other side of the world with my feet sloshing around in the pristine tropical water felt liberating almost beyond description. I of course hadn't expected that a plane trip to a foreign land would magically cure me. All I'd aimed to experience was some modicum of escape — to mentally run away from this illness, even if only for a little while. And although I'd set off on this romantic quest find myself, while standing on that beach I discovered that what I actually wanted to do was lose myself completely.

Disconnected from both the past and the future, I was at last completely lost in the moment. Standing on a picturesque crescent-shaped white-sand beach with only a narrow opening

visible straight ahead imparting a glimpse of the sprawling tropical Andaman Sea, I felt the ever-present tension and anxiety
that had come with CFS begin to drain out of me and drift off
into the ocean. Although the illness itself, unfortunately, hadn't
gone anywhere, the "real world" and all the stress that came
with it definitely had. I felt akin to Leonardo DiCaprio's character in *The Beach* (which, incidentally, was filmed on the exact
spot I happened to find myself crying on), just another naive
traveler in Thailand who, even though they didn't know
precisely what it was, knew they were there searching for something more. Just another traveler who felt, at least for a moment,
that they might've found exactly what they'd been looking for.

In this new free-spirited world, all the ways that this illness
slowed me down didn't seem to matter as much anymore. I
could spend as many days as I needed in various hostels and
guesthouses resting in bed, and with all my moving around and
no one ever bearing witness to or tallying up my downtime, it
somehow didn't seem to count. With its astounding ability to
virtually render my CFS symptoms powerless, backpacking
quickly became a highly addictive drug for me. As long as I was
hopping around the globe, I thought I could hold onto at least
this fragmented version of escape from my illness. While
perpetually on vacation, CFS was manageable and took a back-
seat to what I considered "living" at the time. In fleeing the
responsibilities of *reality* I'd managed a partial escape. Here, I
wasn't my mother or my husband's ex-wife. Here in this back-
packer paradise, my 50 percent improvement was almost
enough. Illness still had me firmly in its clutches, but my prison
cell had increased in size exponentially, and I even felt like I
might have been furloughed.

With this newfound feeling of freedom and adventure, I
was suddenly happier than I'd ever been in my life.

But if travel was my drug of choice, then Canada was

simply poison. I *never* wanted to go back. Yes, Canada represented all the illness and struggle and grief that I desperately wanted to leave behind for good. But it also represented a trap of conventional living that I'd felt I'd fallen into while there, and if I returned might never manage to escape that again as well. The thought of going back to some job that I hated, getting married again, and spending weekends carting my hypothetical kids to soccer games and dance lessons now sounded not just mundane, but unimaginably horrific. I never again wanted to be a slave to my lawn, so effectively and ridiculously domesticated by my grass. In fleeing Canada I'd believed I'd found a loophole. A life hack. As long as I didn't go back, then I'd beaten the system. As long as I didn't go back, then this escape and the dream I was living would never end.

My bliss-filled days quickly turned into weeks, and my budding love affair with Southeast Asia continued to grow. While Australia's mild but stubborn winter lingered, I decided I would cross a couple of Thailand's borders and see what else Asia might have in store. With a venerable treasure trove of countries available a mere seven-dollar bus ride away, Australia could definitely wait.

Despite my physical limitations, I managed to make my way through seven different countries in Southeast Asia, then finally Australia, and then even on to India. I surprised myself with how much sightseeing I was able to pull off, but one thing I never even dreamed of trying to do was to keep up with the pack of energetic travelers around me. There would be no mountain hikes or bicycle safaris or full-day city excursions for me. To the spritely teenage gap-year travelers I would fall in with occasionally, I imagined it seemed conceivable that a decrepit old person in their thirties like myself would have trouble keeping up. And I'd figured that I'd needed a break from talking about being sick almost as much as the world probably needed a break from hearing about it, so I stuck to my made-up excuses for not partaking in the more intense activities and resolved to never mention my chronic illness to anyone. In this bizarre new nomadic life that I was living, CFS was surprisingly easy to hide. And even though I was still definitely sick, because I never talked about CFS it sometimes felt like the illness wasn't even there.

As my travels persisted and my bank balance rapidly approached zero, I happily whipped out my credit cards in service of keeping this epic escape going as long as possible. I found that going into debt to keep my travels afloat was alarmingly easy to rationalize. Just about everyone I knew was in debt, usually for things like home renovations or university tuition, and I reasoned that escaping crippling despair while seeing the world was at least as good of a reason to go into debt as a finished basement was. Each rickety bus or rusty train I boarded headed for yet another unknown and exhilarating destination to explore was another hit of the world's most powerful drug for me, and each time I did it my financial irresponsibility became all the more ingrained and normalized. From the temples and rainforests of Southeast Asia, to the harbors and botanical gardens of Australia, and finally the mausoleums and beaches of India, my credit cards and I managed to keep this backpacking escape going for almost one full year.

As the end of that year approached, with my dwindling credit I secured a one-month rental for a dirt-cheap hut on a tiny Thai tropical island. Although I'd loved every single place that I'd visited, Thailand definitely held a certain allure, so I'd decided to make my way back to where it all started. I was virtually tapped out, and this perpetual vacation of sorts was going to soon have to come to an end. It seemed the ideal spot to relax for a bit while I worked on figuring out my next move.

Only a few days into my island stay, suddenly the only thing that mattered to me was getting my head back above water. Not financially — somehow I wasn't all that stressed about the money yet — but literally. My breaths, rapid and shallow, felt impossible to catch up with. The sea was all around me, salty and formidable and exerting its force against my entire body, all while taunting me and tapping into every primal survival instinct I had. No matter how many gulps of air I sucked in, I still felt as if I were suffocating. *There isn't enough air,* I'd desperately thought to myself. *Why can't I breathe?!*

For once, it wasn't the CFS making me feel this way. And I probably wasn't actually anywhere close to drowning either. What was happening was that I thought I had found my Plan B. I was going to be a scuba diving instructor.

The water and nearby beach were packed with students and diving instructors alike, and as my heart rate slowly decelerated and my panic began to subside after my latest dive, I was able to take stock of the diverse range of accents coming from the scuba professionals around me. One instructor bellowing at her class on the beach was clearly from Germany, and another bobbing on the surface nearby definitely sounded French. Every one of these foreigners with their sun-streaked hair and tanned easy-going faces had managed to escape their home country and live right here on this textbook tropical island and make this glorious Thai beach their office.

I somehow needed to make some money to keep this escape going. So clearly the solution to all my problems was to spend a bunch more money that I didn't have. And with that newfound clarity and this solidly rational plan, I promptly extend the lease on my tiny hut and got busy buying equipment and training for my new career.

The fact that I experienced panic attacks underwater should have been my first clue that there might be something wrong with this plan, but honestly, the ocean trying to drown me didn't hold a candle to the horrors that I was sure awaited me back home in Canada. I was still sick, of course, but I'd decided that I would just get the credentials that I needed to start working on this island, and somehow everything would just be ok. *Maybe you're capable of more than you think you are. You haven't tried to work in almost a year; it will be so much better this time! Look how great you've done this last year! You'll totally be fine. If you want to make it work badly enough, you will find a way.*

The only explanation I have for this ludicrous and naive thinking is my tireless denial. I suspect that because I'd not been talking about my CFS and had pretended for the better part of a year that I was fine, I'd partially convinced myself of this as well. *Overseas Raelan* was a whole new animal — one impervious to obstacles and capable of anything. One way or another, I would make it work.

A few months and a few thousand dollars' worth of training and diving equipment later, I was a competent and skilled (and thankfully no longer hydrophobic) scuba instructor. I had a hobby I adored, but sadly, no new career. Having never actually asked too many questions about salaries, I'd neglected to figure out beforehand that I'd have to work nine days a week to have any hope of making ends meet. And although a scuba diving hobby (once you get the hang of it) is relatively easy-going, the professional end of things required seemingly endless hours spent stocking boats and carrying heavy equipment. This was serious business — so serious that my CFS-riddled body unfortunately just could not keep up with it for more than a couple days a week.

As I sat on the cozy front porch of my little island bungalow and stared at my laptop, I slowly waded through the mess that was my financial life. As I cursed my credit card statement filled with my irresponsible scuba equipment purchases, an email notification popped up on my screen with a subject line that instantly grabbed my attention. It would seem that the supervisor of the NGO (nonprofit organization that operates independently of any government) at which I'd volunteered for a couple months earlier on in my trip while in Phnom Penh, Cambodia had just resigned, and they were wondering if I would be interested in taking on a paid position with them working as her replacement.

Hello, Plan C.

As I read and reread that e-mail I marveled at the unfathomable power of the all-knowing Universe and its ability to put the perfect opportunities in my path just when I needed them. Although intensely beautiful, this tiny Thai tropical island that I'd been living on had started to feel suffocatingly small, and the idea of being in an energetic city like Phnom Penh sounded like a welcome change of pace. And what meaningful work I'd be doing! Social work jobs in this region were few and far between, and here one had pretty much just fallen into my lap exactly when I needed it.

"As you know, here in Cambodia we work mostly in US dollars, and the salary for this position will be US$700 per month," the NGO manager proudly announced during my subsequent Skype interview. "We've just increased it! Your predecessor was only making $450."

Wait. *What?*

Trying my hardest to hide my shock and disappointment at having just been offered what was likely the only worse paying job than my two-days-a-week scuba career, I squeaked out, "Um, with all due respect, I have to ask how I could possibly live on that?"

"Oh, you can rent a room in a house in this neighborhood for very cheap," the interviewer excitedly assured me. "And if you eat the local street food you'll be just fine. It's all about helping the children, right? The last person who held this position refused any pay raises because she didn't want to take any money that could be going to the kids."

Prior to coming to live at this NGO-run center, the Cambodian children this man spoke about had lived in tents on the city's municipal garbage dump — a location they'd chosen for its proximity to the trash hopefully speckled with small items they might be able to sell or trade for food. These children had already endured more adversity and hardship in their short lives than most of us will experience in a lifetime. *Of course* it was all about these kids. Who on earth could say no to this?

"I'm sorry, sir, thank you so much for this opportunity, but I'm going to have to decline."

It turns out I could.

I so wish that I could've told you that the rest of this story was going to be about how I chose to selflessly help these innocent children in need. How altruism won and as a result I helped change the trajectory of some very deserving people's lives for the better. I wanted so very much to do the valuable and noble work of serving severely impoverished children. And even more than that, I wanted to be *thought of* as the type of person who would do such valuable and noble work.

But in reality, this part of my story is about how I wanted Starbucks. And my own place. And pedicures. And the occasional trip to Bali. And above all, I wanted *freedom*, and as much as those kids deserved every bit of help I could give them, this opportunity unfortunately felt very much to me like just another prison.

In that moment I learned an unpleasant but valuable lesson about who I was and who I was not. I was no Mother Teresa. I wasn't even anyone remotely close. I was someone who, despite being desperate to not return to Canada, because she still had some room left on her line of credit felt she'd rather search for more appealing options. It's tough looking at yourself in the mirror for a while after you've just chosen a cup of coffee over helping starving children. But I suspect it would have been even tougher signing up for a life that I knew I wasn't prepared to actually live. I'd tried that before and ended up fantasizing about people dying just so that I could make my escape. These children deserved better than that. These children deserved more than me. More than someone who was sick and unreliable and apparently, at that moment, mostly just in it for the paycheck.

Enter Plan D.

"Yes, of course I have experience with making lesson plans," I lied to the kind older British man on the other end of my Skype interview. "I have teaching experience from a number of different jobs I've held in the past. So creating my own curriculum will be no problem for me."

In reality I had *zero* teaching experience and not a clue what a lesson plan was much less how to make one, but with each passing day I needed money more and more urgently, so I decided that I if I could somehow manage to land a teaching job I would figure out how to actually do it. A friend of a friend had a connection, and it was likely the best opportunity at employment in this region that I was going to get. Although the salary at this international school in Malaysia was still quite modest, it would be enough to keep my snobby Starbucks mug filled.

On the morning of my first day on the job, I hovered over the hallway trash bin on the way to my first class and almost tossed up my breakfast. I had a double period with thirty adolescents waiting for me and absolutely no idea what I was doing. Poetry, I was told, was that day's lesson, and I was supposed to somehow teach these teenagers about a Shakespeare play that I'd never even heard of — never mind understood.

By the afternoon of that first day, CFS had already reared its ugly head, and I'd already hit my energy limit. I had no idea teaching could be so exhausting. It was like staging a six-hour performance where you played all the parts.

"I really could use some caffeine," I mentioned to the woman diligently marking papers next to me in the teacher's lounge. "Is there coffee anyplace here?"

"Only local tea in the box by the wall," she replied without looking up from her grading. "Your best bet for actual coffee is the 7-11 store down the street, but good luck getting the principal's permission to leave the premises during school hours."

Challenge accepted.

Since my exhaustion was far stronger than my fear, I braved this domineering woman's office in service of my desperately needed caffeine fix.

"Do you have a class right now?" she demanded of me as if I were a child and couldn't be trusted to make sound decisions on my own. "You can't go if you have a class."

Duh.

"No class! I'm free until third period," I assured her. "I promise I won't be gone long."

After some hesitation and a couple more unsuccessful attempts at finding a reason to thwart my plans, she admitted defeat and let me go. CFS had shaped me into an unstoppable force when it came to busting through the barriers between me and caffeine, and it was going to take a lot more than this stern-faced woman with too much lipstick to stop me.

Eventually I learned to bring my own super-sized thermos of rocket fuel to work with me, but regardless most of my days still felt like some version of that first one — desperate attempts to find the energy to keep going while battling against my new warden's rigid expectations.

At the end of every day, I'd collapse at home at my apartment and spend every minute away from work trying to recover enough to go back. The nightly handfuls of sleeping pills I took to help me get the rest I so desperately needed got bigger and bigger, and the morning coffees in my enormous thermos got stronger and stronger, and yet the sick leave days I had to take every now and then when I absolutely, positively could not make it through the day just kept piling up more and more.

It was brutal. I was a terrible employee, I had no social life, and I was miserable. But nothing was worse than the fate of being forced to return back to Canada, so I kept on popping my pills and filling my mug and faking my way through *Hamlet*.

For one reason or another many of the teachers were struggling with their jobs at this school, and I'll admit that my misery very much loved the company. "We should come at night and vandalize this place," one of my disgruntled teacher friends joked one afternoon while she and I blew off some steam while eating our lunch in the school cafeteria. She too had had her fair share of humiliating scoldings from the principal and was more than a little fed up. "Or better yet, set it on fire!"

With my mountains of grading perpetually waiting for me and parent-teacher interviews looming ahead, leaving didn't feel like an option, so a blazing inferno seemed like a feasible alternative to escape the predicament in which I found myself. For the rest of that day, I was lost in fantasies about the weathered timbers of my newfound prison burning bright and being razed to the ground. Despite my best attempts at escape, here I was living yet another desperate life where someone dying or something burning down was the only path to happiness I could envision. This whole working experiment was failing miserably, and I had no idea what to do.

But then that night — hand to God — whether through luck or fate or pyrokinesis, while empty that school actually caught on fire, and I never had to go back to that job again.

"Yes, of course I have corporate experience," I lied to the trendily dressed Mr. Plan E sitting across the table from me in my interview. "I've had to hold my own while dealing with the inflated egos of the moguls in a number of different jobs I've held in the past. That will be no problem for me."

In reality I had even less corporate experience than teaching experience (since I once had actually gone to school) and had never met a single mogul (except the kind on a ski slope), but since I was paying my rent with one credit card and paying that one off with another, I knew that I absolutely had to get this job and then somehow figure it out. With the flexible working hours and occasional work-from-home setup that this job offered, I was convinced *this* was absolutely the best opportunity for employment I was going to get.

Even though my recent return to work had been such a catastrophic failure, I knew I needed to avoid my dreaded Canada life at all costs. And after all, this job was vastly different than the teaching one, so I just *knew* it would be a vastly different experience from that last blazing catastrophe. *That job was just so hectic,* I told myself. *This job is so much slower paced than being a teacher. I'm sure I'll be ok.*

The flexible working arrangements did allow me to keep my head above water — but just barely. Since I was pretty sure that chronic illness was not one of the more sought-after qualities in an employee, I didn't tell a soul at this company about my having CFS. Even though I could mostly work from home, it was still incredibly difficult for me to pull it all off, and it wasn't ever — even for one day — easy.

But the in-office meetings that I had to attend (and often facilitate) were going to be the death of me. They left me completely depleted. As a result, I was sick and exhausted all the time while always working so hard to try to hide it. I *hated* lying about it all, but I didn't feel I had any other choice.

"I've got the flu," I would sheepishly mutter to my boss. "I'm not going to be able to make it in today."

"Didn't you have the flu last week?" he would ask, sounding slightly skeptical and more than a little confused. "Or was that the eye infection?"

"No, that was food poisoning," I'd lie while trying to sound convincing and confident in my answer. "Bad chicken from the food court. The eye infection was the week before."

A few months into working this job, while collapsed on the grey Ikea throw rug on the living room floor of my modest downtown apartment, I felt my body betray me for the zillionth time. *I see another "eye infection" in my immediate future,* I facetiously thought to myself. My eyes, of course, were fine. But expecting my boss to understand that the five minutes of light exercise I'd just done on my apartment floor would have me bed-bound tomorrow was kind of a big ask.

Despite having mostly maintained the same mediocre state of health for years, I never stopped believing that eventually I would absolutely 100 percent recover from CFS. With my fridge perpetually stocked with grilled chicken breasts and pre-portioned raw vegetable snacks, I strove to give my body the fuel it needed to carry out some small amounts of physical activity. But no matter what I tried, my body always crashed in spectacular fashion.

I knew of course that the stress that all these failed attempts caused was in no way conducive to healing. Exercise — no matter how little — always came with a hefty price tag. But despite the years' worth of evidence strongly suggesting that any attempts at physical activity would always make me worse, I just wouldn't give up. Sometimes I'd get far enough with my exercise regimen to start seeing some small improvements, but without fail I'd always eventually crash hard and be forced to abandon my efforts yet again.

And to make matters worse, I also often *did* get actual food poisoning, eye infections, and the flu. My immune system was in such bad shape and my fake excuses were so mingled up with reality that even I started having a tough time discerning the lies from the truth.

Before I got sick with CFS, should any one string of support in my life be cut, there were a thousand others that were still holding me in place. With CFS, I lived my life perpetually hanging by a single string. Every single time I pushed myself and tried to work on improving my health, I was gambling on that one already overtaxed thread to continue holding me up. It was a horrible way to live, and even now I cringe just thinking about how grueling those times living in *survival mode* were for me. I was always struggling and constantly felt like I was faking my way through my life. Somehow I got by, but it was absolutely no way to live. Despite the partial escape from suffering that I'd managed by escaping Canada, it was still a far cry from being free.

6

LAST CHANCE FOR FREEDOM

Sitting on my new balcony, gazing out at the juxtaposed cityscape of the modern high-rises and rickety slums of Jakarta, I felt my body relax and my shoulders drop a good six inches. What I felt in that moment after having just arrived in Indonesia was reminiscent of that same unencumbered feeling I'd experienced years ago when I'd first arrived in Southeast Asia and found myself gleefully splashing around in Thailand on Leonardo DiCaprio's picture-perfect beach. Once again — this time amongst the racket and chaos typical of an over-crowded developing city — I took a moment to observe the dissolving stress and toxicity that, with this most recent move, I'd once again managed to enjoy.

With this latest escape — I'll admit — I had an accomplice. How I'd ever found the energy to spare to date is still beyond me, but loneliness, as they say, is a powerful motivator. For the longest time, despite my best efforts at finding *The One*, not one of the men who would sit across from me at the restaurant dinner table had ever even earned the privilege of a first name in subsequent correspondence or conversation with friends.

When sharing the stories of those mostly laughable first, second, and extremely rare third dates, nicknames would be conferred for their comedic value (or sometimes even sarcastic revenge for those particularly bad dates).

Buddha Beads, for example, earned his moniker not only because this Aussie donned a particular type of prayer necklace on our first date, but also for my having to explain to him what these beads were actually used for. There was also *Mr. Chivalry,* a Scot who, upon discovering (at the same time as me) that I'd recently been pickpocketed, and hence he would have to pay for our drinks, proceeded to down *both* of our beers himself before picking up the check and making a speedy exit. And of course *Mr. Buthisface* because, um, well . . . once you take the not-so-appealing head off this German — yum!

As the lonely months dragged on, my hopes of finding someone whose name I would bother remembering were dwindling just as rapidly as the options worth swiping right on my dating app were. Even with virtually every single man (and probably quite a few married ones) available for me to shop through and select with just the touch of a button, I somehow couldn't find anyone whom I deemed worthy of what little energy I had to spare.

Until *The American,* who because of his sharp (and well-informed) fashion sense, his insistence on not only paying for our drinks but also retrieving mine and hand-delivering it to me, and his hunky head that absolutely should remain fastened to the rest of his body at all times, left me no option but to actually take note of his real name and use it when referring to him: *Geoffrey.* With his quick wit, engaging conversation skills, and stunning good looks, he swiftly made me forget *Mr. Jorts, The Flosser,* and *The Italian Non-Stallion.* Lost in our romantic sea of candlelit dinners, sun-drenched afternoons chillaxing by the pool, and tropical island paradise weekend getaways, it was game over for us. So when his job eventually sent him to Indonesia, it was a no-brainer for me to pack up my mountain of scuba gear and go with him.

I think for quite some time I'd been waiting for someone to save me. Those past few years I'd felt as if I'd been drowning, and no matter how much I splashed and flailed around I never seemed to be able to learn how to swim. While acting as my own savior I'd found myself wanting. Lacking. Unequipped and incapable of getting the job done.

Since I'd never before met anyone in my life who was capable of saving me, I'm not sure why I ever held out hope for this possibility. Any past relationships that I'd had, for the most part, had only dragged me further down. But this time, things seemed different. There was a level of maturity in my relationship with Geoffrey that I'd never before known was possible, and with that maturity came a supportive and equal playing field that made exciting and fantastic things seem possible.

In this new and solid relationship of equals, I finally understood and internalized the significant distinction between the act of *empowerment* and that of *saving*. That the one-sided expectation of saving should never be put on anyone, and that the only person who could and should save me was me. That with the right support, I was unbelievably powerful and so incredibly capable of saving myself all on my own. His only job in this department was to help me hold a mirror up so that I could see when the patterns that I'd created for myself were not working. And in thanks, I was to help him hold that same mirror up to himself and help him see the same.

By this point I was starting to forget what a life without constant struggle even felt like. Not a single day since I'd first gotten sick all those years ago had been easy. Not a single day had passed without some kind of battle required to get through it. After almost ten years of living with chronic illness, I knew I was ready to finally put this disease behind me for good. It's not that I hadn't tried in the past, and it's not that only with the love a good man would I succeed. It was a process of maturing and achieving some hard-won wisdom that I was able to see with complete clarity that I was going to get better this time. With my reflective mirror in hand and those supportive strings firmly back in place, this was it. There would be no more messing around. No more getting only partway there. I was *done* with being trapped by my illness and resolved to grab those keys dangling in front of me and free myself from this jailhouse called CFS once and for all.

I labeled the digital folder on my laptop *FREEDOM*. All caps — because I wanted that sentiment screamed at me every single time I opened it. As I clicked through the documents stored inside and admired all the planning and hard work I'd already done, I tried to figure out if I was missing anything. *Diet plan?* Check. *Exercise regimen?* Check. *Daily journal? Fasting schedule? Detox checklist?* Check. Check. Check.

Thankfully, from my years of experimenting, I'd actually learned a lot about healing and what worked with CFS for me. I'd made some small gains along the way, but had never found the time or space to keep anything up consistently. In trying everything I would end up really trying nothing. For quite some time I'd felt akin to an overweight person with an effective diet and exercise plan in hand — just no access to healthy food or a gym. But in this new supportive life with Geoffrey in

Jakarta, I had everything I needed to at long last put the final plan in place.

"This might take a while," I hesitantly said to him not too long after I'd moved in. "As determined as I am, CFS is something I've been battling for almost a decade, and I don't think it's going to go away overnight."

His unwavering support always astounded me. With what appeared to be barely a blink of an eye's hesitation, he jumped on board with my plan to get well and volunteered to be the financial backbone of our budding relationship for the duration of that process. "Why don't you set aside this entire year to focus on getting healthy," he casually responded, as if simply offering up his last French fry. "And if it takes longer, no worries."

With his predictably unfaltering wisdom, he was right — this recovery process was definitely going to be a marathon, not a sprint. We had to be mentally prepared for the long haul, and if it ended up taking less than a year, then that would just be a nice bonus for both of us.

With this long-awaited opportunity to heal finally in front of me, I started to fantasize about what life could be like once CFS was no longer holding me down. I imagined posting a picture of myself on Instagram where I'd just busted through the finish line of a marathon, and triumphantly writing the caption "Fuck you, CFS!" below it. I envisioned myself soaking up the sun and battling the punishing ocean waves in Bali while finally learning to surf. I imagined a life where, free from physical limitations, I could pursue any career I wanted — and the stunning beach house that my newfound success might permit me to own. I imagined possibly being able to one day even help others overcome similar struggles. I imagined writing this book.

I also had to change who I was in order to become the person I wanted to be. I realize that sounds dramatic, but if I still had one foot in my past I couldn't put both feet forward on this new path I wanted to take. And so I scanned the emails in my inbox full of invitations for Jakarta expat mingles — boozy events meant to connect foreigners living abroad — and I went through each and clicked on *unsubscribe*. While living in Kuala Lumpur I was the leader for such groups, but with my new dedicated healing regimen I knew that I would not even be able to attend such events as a guest. A social life meant committing my energy to things other than healing, and that was something that for the time being I could not afford to do.

After clearing out the contents of my inbox, the liquor cabinet and pantry were next. I loved gin and can still obsess over a freshly made G&T, but I loved the thought of being healthier more. Any culprit whose ingredient list indicated an alcohol content, displayed the words *refined* or *glucose,* or any word containing more than three syllables, had to go. All the poisons masquerading as cleaners stored under the kitchen sink were also tossed into the trash. No more toxic dryer sheets. No more of Geoffrey's beloved chemical-filled air fresheners. *This is the time for removing nails from my coffin,* I'd adamantly told him, *not putting more in.*

I knew this was my chance, and that opportunities like this, ones where I was able to completely prioritize myself and my health, would not come along again. I think that was the biggest change of all — it really did feel like now or never for me, and I acted like it. If I blew it, or half-assed it in any way, this time would be wasted, and I would never get it back. And I was under no illusions, given my family history, that the conse-quences of that couldn't be severe. I was ready to maintain absolute focus and get myself completely healthy so that I could fully live life again and finally leave behind all of that struggle and pain.

I stopped wanting to get better. *Wanting* was in the past. I *needed* — once and for all — to be free.

But if wanting ain't getting, then neither is needing. In the next chapters I'm going to spell out exactly what it took for me to get better, but to wipe away any lingering illusions about how needing something instead of just wanting it is the key, let me take you inside what it was like.

It was 4:00 a.m. on one fairly typical morning a few months into my healing sabbatical, and as usual, the scalding hot water in the bathtub was making me sweat profusely. On that day, as was typical of most days, in the last twenty-four hours I'd already racked up two baths and one shower. If it weren't for the greasy ponytail on my head clumsily disguising a couple days' worth of dry shampoo, you'd swear I had some sort of compulsion for being clean. What I actually had was a grave issue with some aching muscles. My daily workouts, despite being extremely humble, were putting my body through the wringer.

When it came to the most effective way to spend what energy I had, initially, I'd determined that the best bang for my buck was exercise. And since I couldn't manage much in that department, this meant that 98 percent of my time was a slave to that 2 percent spent doing my measly workouts. After having completed my daily few minutes of lightweight physical activity, the remainder of my days were spent resting up enough to be able to hopefully be able to manage a few more minutes of exercise again the next day.

With my body reeling from the shock of this newly introduced exertion, many mornings I wouldn't be able to pull myself out of bed before noon, and the remainder of the day, aside from small breaks to get some sun, prepare some healthy food, or do some light detoxing activity, were spent curled up with a book or Netflix. The headaches, body aches, and crippling fatigue had me captive. No friends. No hobbies. Just recovery.

But despite all the unpleasantness, I wasn't deterred because I was making progress, and progress, as it turns out, is incredibly addictive. I recognized pretty early on that this year of deprivation in service of my health was going to reap rewards far greater than any suffering experienced or sacrifices made. After just a few disciplined months of following my healing plan, the results were already undeniable. It was no longer optimism or rose-colored glasses enabling me to believe that I was getting well — it was a cold hard assessment of the facts.

My recovery plan encompassed four areas: nutrition, exercise, emotional well-being, and overall body healing support. Despite sounding fairly straightforward, it often wasn't. Healing from CFS was definitely an iterative process, and as the months passed I learned far more about what was required to get healthy than I'd known when I'd first gotten started.

My diet, for instance, for a long time was all wrong. And as a result, for the first few months the progress I saw with my health was incredibly slow going. But once I got my nutritional plan tweaked to perfection, my progress came in leaps and bounds. Seriously — with just this one change I started witnessing the dramatic, night-and-day kind of changes that, upon hearing about them, most people think you're making up.

It was absolutely astounding what a difference eating the right foods made. Research shows that depending on what you consume you can get better or worse from eating just one meal. And initially I ate months' worth of the wrong meals! Oh, the progress I could have made had I eaten properly from the start.

Throughout this process I paid very close attention to what was going on with my body. If at any time it felt like I wasn't making progress, or worse, that I was going backward, I took the time to examine what was happening. If I suddenly felt worse, I'd first allow myself a moment to feel sorry for myself and wallow in the injustice of it all. After years of suffering, my tolerance for CFS was definitely wearing thin. After a pause to acknowledge that being sick was frustrating and depressing and that it was ok to not love this part of the process, I would then go into full-on detective mode. *Is my diet different? Am I under more stress? What in my behavior or routine has recently been different? Could this simply be the flu?*

I no longer wrote suffering off as something that just happens; I examined it closely and acted accordingly. And more often than not, I could find the culprit and rectify the situation.

Maybe most importantly, I also discovered that that internal voice that would sometimes tell me that I was failing was a liar. A bad day or week did not equal failure. Bad days were a part of the process and I learned to expect and accept them as an inevitable part of my healing journey.

Despite it not being easy, my CFS healing plan was, in the end, simple in its design. And as I stayed the course, my energy levels slowly increased, my endurance improved, and my overall feeling of well-being just got better. After years of living life with an invisible force pulling me back, I finally began to feel this power reverse and begin propelling me forward instead. Slowly, I got to stop being afraid of life. Afraid of pushing too hard. Afraid I wouldn't have the energy to last through the birthday party or the errand-running or the company dinner. And most importantly, I got to stop being afraid that the people around me would finally get fed up with all my limitations and leave me behind for good.

Instead, I began feeling excited. Excited to experience workouts with no limits. Excited to rejoin that whole world of activities such as hiking and swimming that had for so long been off-limits. Excited to finally hold my head up high and share this active and vibrant version of myself with the people I loved. Excited to imagine a life spent with Geoffrey that didn't involve compromises because of my health.

Seeing such results without having any surgeries or taking any prescription medications or supplements for healing flew in the face of what Western medicine had always led me to believe was possible. But as time marched on it was undeniable — my healing plan was working and I was getting better.

I didn't know it at the time, but I'd created a program for myself for healing from CFS that falls under an emerging mainstream medicine practice called *lifestyle medicine*. In their book *Undo It!* Dean Ornish, MD, and Anne Ornish explain how using this peer-reviewed and scientifically backed approach to healing — using simple yet powerful lifestyle changes to reverse the progression of common chronic diseases — is incredibly powerful. Our bodies, these authors explain, often have a remarkable capacity to begin healing, and much more quickly than we had once believed. Often our biggest obstacle is the skepticism that such simple lifestyle changes can have such powerful, far-reaching, measurable improvements — and how fast you can feel better.

When we're sick, we've been trained to seek out specific remedies that will work for our particular illness and our illness alone. We actually don't seem to want our bodies to heal themselves (as they so expertly do in the right conditions); we want a doctor to write us a prescription that will. We expect there to be a specific medication or treatment tailored to each and every illness that exists. It feels wrong somehow that something that falls under the general heading of something like *lifestyle medicine* could be what will heal us. As if this diminishes the severity of our condition somehow and makes it less legitimate. But just because the treatment isn't 100 percent unique, it doesn't mean that the illness isn't. The reality is that there are general things that we can do that will go a long way toward healing many illnesses.

In the end, it actually ended up taking me a little longer than a year to reach my goal, but I finally did reach it. After almost two years of dedication to my healing regimen, I did in fact 100 percent recover from CFS. Two years might sound like a long time to some, but that time gained me an untold number of years to come where I get to live fully and be free from the horrible restraints of chronic illness. Those two years were, beyond any shadow of a doubt, the most productive years of my life. People spend much longer than that on university degrees and other similar endeavors with much smaller rewards waiting for them at the finish line. For me, putting in only a couple of years of focused work to gain my freedom back was a no-brainer. And had I had this book when I started, it likely wouldn't even have taken me that long.

Despite my spectacular end results, I unfortunately can't say that the entire experience was all this beautiful process of becoming one with my body and marveling at how it flourished when I supported its healing efforts. Some weeks were definitely like that, but many weren't. It was always clear that CFS wasn't going to go away without a fight. At times, just when I'd think that I'd gotten past some aspect of CFS, that I'd found the formula to remedy this specific piece of my struggle, I'd find myself back where I started, having to start that fight all over again. I was in a battle to get my life back, my freedom back, and at times there wasn't anything beautiful or serene about it. I'm definitely not in any way claiming that fully recovering from CFS was easy. What I am saying is that, thankfully, for me it was possible.

Fortunately, my second time around of seriously trying to get well was a completely different experience than the first time.

Despite my unshakable motivation, this still wasn't always a flawless journey spent in a pristine bubble of healing. It was far from perfect. Life, as it does, threw some small kinks into my plan here and there. I just did the best I could to minimize how much those bumps slowed me down. I made mistakes, and I certainly wasn't always a role model with my behavior. But for the most part, I stayed on track, and when I didn't, I figured out how to get back on track quickly.

I've also learned that expecting too much of myself can be unrealistic, even a bit cruel. I didn't always get everything right. No one could. I just made sure that as time went on, I learned how to get it wrong less often. I learned how to better cope with the backslides in my health and bounce back quicker. I learned how to do damage control and to never ever forget that pain is information that is there to show me how to tweak my plan and further speed up my recovery.

During the tough times, acknowledging and celebrating the small steps that I'd made in the right direction gave me the boost I needed to keep pushing through. I made sure to give myself tons of credit for how hard I was working and to give myself huge pats on the back for coming as far as I had. I celebrated myself, my efforts, and my progress all the time. After a decade of suffering, I knew that each and every seemingly small step in the direction toward good health was actually huge.

Knowing what I know now, it makes me a bit frustrated and sad that it took me so long to put all the pieces together and finally get well. By not having the right information from the start, I ended up wasting so much time and suffering so much more than was necessary. It shouldn't have taken me anywhere near ten years to get better. In fact, it needn't have even taken me the two years that it did when I buckled down again in the end. But I did the best I could with the information I had at the time.

In the next four parts, I'm going to spell out exactly what I did that allowed me to finally, once and for all, completely recover from chronic fatigue syndrome. I hope these next chapters and the keys to healing that worked so well for me might be a companion for you too as you find your own healing path. As a layperson, all I can do is share my experience. I'm sharing what worked for me, and it will be up to you and your doctor to determine what might work best for you.

It's good to take charge of our bodies and take some initiative in determining our own healing plan, but finding a doctor that you trust and respect to discuss things with before trying them is important as well. The doctor might not always get it right, but they're one more person you have on your team to help you make informed decisions as you go.

Just keep in mind that not all doctors are created equal. When you meet with a doctor, if that doctor is telling you that nothing can be done, if that doctor is telling you that this is all in your head, or if that doctor just wants to manage your symptoms and is not actively helping you cure yourself of this disease, then *find another doctor.*

Doctors can't do everything, and they certainly can't cure everyone. Your doctor is only human. And not even a superhuman — just a regular old human. Expecting any one person to know everything, to never make mistakes, and to be the single source of truth would be an incredibly unfair expectation to put on anyone, doctors and laymen alike. What doctors *can* do is work with us, even when they don't know the answers. They can teach us to take charge of our health and to learn as much as we can about our own body and its unique needs. They can guide us and be skilled and knowledgeable consultants for us as we experiment and try different things. They can and should be our supportive health allies, here to assist us in making informed decisions about what to do next.

In these next chapters, you won't find a bunch of regurgitated research on the existing healing modalities for this illness. What I have found in the literature that has helped me I have most certainly included here, but for the most part, what the various experts out there have had to say about this disease regrettably hasn't helped me much. I suspect you're in the same boat as well, and if that's the case then I hope you find what you are looking for here.

The process of reaching our goals is rarely luck — it's strategy. I worked hard, I experimented like crazy, and I found the strategies that worked. In the end, just a few simple and rigorous lifestyle changes led to massive breakthroughs for me, and I hope they help you elude the grip of our captor as well.

IV

FINDING FREEDOM
WITH FOOD

7

GATHERING YOUR HEALING FUEL

There's no escaping it: what we put into our bodies will always have a big impact on our health and how we feel. And why would we want to escape it? Food is awesome! Yes, even the stuff that is good for you.

Eating well seems like it should be straightforward, but with the insane amount of conflicting information floating around out there, for a long time I was quite confused. Actually, I'm still a bit confused about what is generally considered good food for the average non-CFS person. Have you ever watched any of those videos where a panel of *experts* have a discussion about what people should and shouldn't be eating? No one seems to agree, and it's enough to make your head explode.

The food industry is a massive business, and in its relentless money-making pursuit it's concocted all sorts of food options that can appear healthy but in reality are anything but. There are also so many food plans out there, each one insisting that its way is the best and only way to go. Some use points, some count calories. Others focus on how many fats or carbohydrates we consume. Some tell us to monitor our body's pH levels or to eat according to our blood type. Some insist we must eat meat. Others proclaim that a vegan diet is the only path to health. There really is a mess of information out there, and it can be so incredibly easy to get lost in it all.

I don't think there will ever be a one-size-fits-all plan for nutrition. We are all beautifully unique, and what makes our own bodies thrive will vary somewhat. But when it comes to recovering from CFS, I've definitely found that in my experience there are some **specific things** you can do that can catapult you toward becoming healthy. There *is* something happening in the body of a person with CFS, which tells me that the fuel we give that body can be vital to recovering from it.

Since what goes into my body is extremely important, I don't want to waste vital space on my plate with foods that aren't helping me stay strong and achieve all my health goals. I no longer make compromises when it comes to my diet. I've realized the costs of eating the wrong things, and those costs are so much greater than I ever realized.

When it comes to disease, people place a lot of the blame on genetics, but Dr. Michael Gregor, author of *How Not to Die,* insists that the most harmful thing we inherit from our families is actually their bad habits, especially around food. So the good news is, even if you've been dealt a bad genetic deck, you can still reshuffle it with diet.

Again, we are all likely a bit unique in this regard, but if I could dial back the clock to Day One with CFS, this is what I'd tell myself about how to use nutrition to properly fuel my body and propel me toward freedom from CFS.

First things first, I would tell myself to eat some bugs. I'm talking, of course, about **probiotics**, and not the creepy crawlies hanging out in your backyard. When it comes to nutrition and healing from CFS, this is the absolute best place to start. This is the glue that holds everything else together. If your microbiome (the community of micro-organisms living in your gut) isn't in order, nothing else will fall into place.

When most people think about probiotics (if they think about them at all), they think about supplements. Over the years I've spent literally *thousands* of dollars on probiotic supplements. I took them by the handful in an attempt to flood my gut with good bacteria in the hopes that these good bugs would go to battle against the *bad guys* and help me restore my health. But no matter how many bottles I plowed through, I never noticed any improvements in my health. In time, tired of feeling like I was wasting my money, I eventually stopped taking them.

Then one day I stumbled across a book called *The Diet Myth: The Real Science Behind What We Eat* written by Tim Spector, a professor of genetic epidemiology and a reputable scientist specializing in the study of diet and how it affects our microbiome. In his book, Spector details how eating a high-fiber diet along with foods naturally rich in good bacteria is the key to attaining and maintaining a healthy gut.

After reading his book I understood why supplements weren't working and why natural foods would. Not to make a long story short, but in supplement form the probiotics were likely dead, whereas in their natural state they were alive and kickin'. When we try and heal our gut by popping pills it just doesn't seem to do much good. So I immediately got to work looking for ways to incorporate more foods naturally rich in live probiotics into my diet. I started off with some store-bought fermented foods like soft cheeses and kefir. It was a start, but I wasn't sure if these were the best choices. Plus, the store-bought options were expensive, and I could never really be sure about their quality.

The more I learned about fermented foods, the more I realized how simple and easy they were to make at home. I learned how to make my own sauerkraut and other fermented vegetables, then kombucha, and finally kefir. Before long, with all my home fermentation practices, I'd eliminated the need to buy the pricey store-made products completely.

Fermented foods quickly became a regular part of my meals, and I could not believe the benefits I saw from adding them to my diet. The changes in my body were significant and undeniable. I really just could not get over how much my body improved once I started this practice.

The most immediate change I saw after taking in lots of probiotic bacteria in food form was with my bathroom time. For years I'd dealt with recurrent and painful bouts of constipation. Getting my microbiome in good shape made these struggles almost completely a thing of the past. I know this isn't a very sexy topic, but seriously, are there many things more satisfying in life than regular and healthy bowel movements? I think not.

Actually, come to think of it, consuming probiotic-rich foods eliminated virtually every unsexy problem I had. Once I started flooding my body with good bacteria, I also eliminated all cases of urinary tract infections, vaginal yeast infections, and hemorrhoids — three things that before this had unfortunately made regular appearances in my life. Once I was eating a diet rich in fiber and healthy bacteria, all these issues completely disappeared for good.

With the addition of the probiotic-rich foods to my diet, my health overall just got better too. My immune system was much stronger, and I got sick with colds and flus so much less often. I was less bloated, and overall everything in my body just seemed to function better.

I also stopped having issues with food control. Even if there were no other benefits from eating probiotic-rich food (which there definitely are), this one right here would be more than reason enough for me to keep up this practice. With so many of us out there battling food cravings and struggling with issues around controlling our food intake, how do more of us not know about this remedy? For years I'd felt like a slave to food, and a ridiculous amount of my energy went into trying to get myself to eat the right things and to stay away from the wrong ones. For most of my life I'd experienced intense food cravings that at times felt bigger than me and almost completely impossible to control.

After I got serious about restoring my intestinal health, I discovered that what I'd chalked up for years as weak willpower was mostly just a result of my body dealing with and responding to an imbalance of microorganisms in my gut, resulting in intense, problematic cravings and chronic issues with over-eating. With the probiotic-rich foods in my diet, I could suddenly keep a chocolate cake sitting in the fridge all week and easily not touch it. Seriously, this former hardcore sugar addict actually forgets the freaking cake even exists. It's really unbelievable that I spent so many years battling food cravings while blaming my weak willpower when all that time the issue was really with my gut.

If you're committed to putting live probiotics into your system, then you probably want to keep them alive once they are inside you. It's pretty obvious by their name why you should avoid antibiotics as much as possible, but I also stopped taking the birth control pill, because these two things essentially will go to war with your intestinal system. By definition an antibiotic can't play nice with probiotics, and in her book *Gut and Psychology Syndrome*, Dr. Natasha Campbell-McBride helped me understand that the contraceptive pill has the same damaging influence on these microorganisms as antibiotics. (Essentially steroids in the pill have an ability to suppress the immune system and change the composition of bodily flora.)

I'd always suspected that probiotics could bring health benefits, but I'd really underestimated the extent to which this was true. And once my body was working better and my food cravings had disappeared, implementing the rest of my healthy eating plan was a piece of cake (uneaten, of course).

If you think probiotics are transformative, then just wait for what's next.

Initially, my healing diet during my recovery consisted of vegetables, fruit, whole grains, nuts, seeds, lean meat, dairy, and eggs. I also supplemented with some whey protein shakes. I kept the starchy food to a minimum and ate virtually zero junk. This seemed to work all right for me, and I definitely made some gains with my health, though I couldn't tell if it was due to what I was eating (or in spite of it). The food I ate felt lean and wholesome, and at the time I thought that this was the best diet for me. But I wasn't close to being back to full health, and my body really struggled to adapt to exercise. For a fitness freak like me that was a sign that there was still room for improvement.

The next big breakthrough I had after getting probiotics into my diet was learning how to **Go Green**. Midway through my recovery I watched a documentary by director Kip

Anderson called *What the Health*, a film depicting the drastic improvements people see in their health after only a couple weeks on a **whole-foods plant-based** (WFPB) diet.[1] You might think that a WFPB diet is a vegan diet, and you'd be right. But WFPB is a *healthy* vegan diet. The WFPB distinction is important because, as this documentary points out, Oreos and Coke are vegan!

This film highlights that although there are definitely some strong carnivorous species out there to be found, some of the largest and strongest animals on the planet are definitely herbivores as well. We've been brainwashed to believe we'll develop some kind of protein deficiency if we don't eat animal products at every meal, and the very sad reality is that this erroneous belief is literally killing us. When people are tested by doctors after switching to a WFPB diet, their vitamin intake and overall nutrition measurably improves.

When we stop eating meat, volume-wise we actually get to start eating *more* food, and when that food is all plant-based, that means we are getting massive quantities and huge varieties of nutrients. Imagine sitting down for breakfast and, in place of that greasy bacon and eggs, you instead find fresh peaches, pears, berries, and pineapple next to a sweet potato and mushroom tofu scramble sprinkled with pistachios and cashews. Come lunchtime you ditch the cheeseburger and fries and instead overload your plate with colorful vegetable dishes packed full of bell peppers, tomatoes, onions, broccoli, and butternut squash, alongside the biggest serving you can manage of a barley, quinoa, or farro stir fry. Add to this some hummus, guacamole, and bean dips to top things off and you've just ingested infinitely more nutrients than those chicken wings or pork chops can ever dream of giving you. And we haven't even gotten to dinner yet!

People worry about not getting all the nutrients they need

while on a plant-based diet, but the fact is that you're likely not getting the nutrition that you need on an animal-based diet.

Notice that I said animal-based diet. When people hear vegan, their first thought is to stop eating meat. But what I want to say to those who are suffering from CFS is that you need to think *bigger* than just meat. For example, I've always thought of eggs as healthy, but this documentary highlighted a study that showed that eating just one egg can be as bad as smoking five cigarettes for life expectancy.[2] While being interviewed for *What the Health*, physician and nutrition expert Dr. Michael Kaper explains that eggs are made up of concentrated saturated fat and cholesterol, which cause all kinds of damage once consumed. He insists there's nothing good at all about eggs and that they have no place in a healthy diet.

Milk is also worrisome. During their interviews in *What the Health*, Dr. Neal Barnard, president of the Physicians Committee for Responsible Medicine and Dr. Michael Gregor, an expert in clinical nutrition, shared something that is probably surprising to many people (myself included). Harvard researchers (among other reputable sources) have debunked the myth that calcium from milk gives us strong bones. There is zero correlation between milk and bone health: in fact, people who drink larger amounts of milk have more bone fractures, higher rates of cancer, and live shorter lives. The reality is that milk products have an opioid-like effect on our brains, keeping us eating them despite the fact that, because of them, we're gaining weight and unhealthier than we've ever been.

And what about cheese? According to Dr. Alan Goldhamer, founder of the TrueNorth Health Center, cheese is one of the single best foods for *compromising* your health that you're going to find. It's an animal product, so you have all the issues that come with the biological concentration of toxins, plus it's highly processed and very high in saturated fat. Dr. Goldhamer insists that no child or adult human needs to eat cheese, or drink the milk of a cow (or a giraffe or a mouse or any other animal) to be healthy. Milk produced by other species isn't "designed" for humans, and we are only doing ourselves a disservice by consuming any products made from it.

And yes, leaving behind an animal-based diet also means leaving behind meat. We're not talking about how decades down the road there will be some consequences if you eat meat. In the documentary Dr. Gregor explains how within minutes of eating it we get a burst of inflammation. It's of course also true that there are long-term health benefits from giving up meat. And Dr. Barnard explains how carcinogens form in any kind of meat as it is cooked, and by far the biggest source of carcinogens are coming from chicken. He insists all meat products are cancer-causing foods and should come with warning labels just as cigarettes do because their contribution to health issues is huge and pervasive.

Please understand that this is not an issue about whether or not the meat, eggs, and dairy you eat are organic. Even in their organic state, they remain a pure animal-based food. But just in case you're wondering, the film does point out just how much of the animal-based food chain relies on antibiotics to survive. In the USA, the pharmaceutical industry sells 80 percent of all the antibiotics that it makes to animal agriculture. Even if we are careful to not abuse antibiotics ourselves, there's just no avoiding them when we are eating animal products.

I don't know how to explain the changes that I saw in my body on the WFPB diet without people thinking that I'm exaggerating or even outright lying. They were nothing short of extraordinary. Although the serious changes in my body took some time, I started noticing some small improvements with my health from the very first day of eating this way.

The first thing I noticed, oddly enough, was that I started sleeping significantly better. And when I woke up I even looked better. As I got older I started noticing that when I'd wake up in the morning my face would be puffy and swollen. It got so bad that I started sleeping on a wedge pillow so that my head would stay elevated and gravity could take the puffiness elsewhere. After only a few days of eating this way, my face was no longer puffy at all. The WFPB foods worked so well at fixing this that I even got to ditch the annoying wedge pillow. After a few months on the WFPB foods I looked like I'd gotten a facelift. I really looked and felt like I was getting younger just because of the foods that I was eating.

The bloating in my abdominal region also went down, making me look leaner and like I'd instantly lost a few pounds. My bathroom time was also a dream. I'd been so impressed to see how much the fermented foods had helped with food digestion and elimination, but with the WFPB diet this whole situation got better than I ever knew it could be.

And despite feeling fairly energetic by this point in my CFS recovery, before switching to the WFPB diet I still had to take a short nap after lunch most days. But with this new diet change I stopped taking naps completely. I was recovering from my workouts so much faster, and the progress I was seeing at the gym was unparalleled to anything else I'd ever experienced. I'm convinced that had I started eating this way from the start, those first months of exercise would have been far easier for me to get through.

Even my menstrual cycle regulated itself into the normal range. Ever since I was a teenager, I'd experienced incredibly irregular periods — at times going six whole months between each cycle. Since this was always how it had been, I'd assumed that this issue was something genetic. It never occurred to me that my menstrual cycles could become normal, and certainly not from simply changing my diet. Now in my forties, I have a regular menstrual cycle for the first time in my life.

Maybe the biggest win was saving money, and I don't mean by not buying meat. Now that I follow a predominantly WFPB diet, my nutritional supplement days are also done. From the tens of thousands of dollars' worth of supplements I've taken over the years, I've never once in my life seen a specific observable improvement from taking a single one of them. In my experience, they have been a complete waste of money. The biggest gains I've always seen in my health have come when I focus on getting my nutrients from food.

If you're serious about getting healthy, in my experience the WFPB diet is absolutely the way to go. Please trust me on this one — as long as food tastes good and makes you feel good, you won't care at all what's in it. I know it sounds restrictive and you think you will be bored with your food options. But once you get serious with it and take your focus off meat, eggs, and dairy, you'll discover a whole new world of options beyond salad and tofu. I didn't even know that tempeh existed or how good smoothie bowls could taste. And you haven't really lived, in my opinion, until you've eaten dragon fruit.

It probably helps that these days the Internet is packed full of delicious healthy vegan recipes, making meal-planning a breeze. Just a couple examples of the ample great options out there are https://deliciouslyella.com and http://www.plantplate.com. This really is a good example of *Don't knock it until you try it*, because I can almost guarantee that most people have the wrong impression about what a healthy vegan diet actually looks and tastes like.

I've heard vegetarians and vegans say things like this before, and to be honest I don't think I ever really believed them. But seriously, I don't miss cooking meat one single bit. I actually found that I liked the WFPB meals *better* than the meat-heavy ones. The plant-based meals I make are so enjoyable that neither Geoffrey (who fell in love with WFPB foods despite not having to) nor I feel like we are missing out on anything at all. Once you make the switch to a WFPB diet you will thoroughly enjoy what you are eating and feel so good about all the nutrients that you see on your plate. You will never feel like you are sacrificing anything by eating this way.

If going all-in sounds too drastic for you, aim for 90 percent WFPB foods instead. By sticking mostly to a WFPB diet you get to enjoy many of the benefits to your health that these foods bring, and by allowing small amounts of animal products in you get to live a life that doesn't feel too rigid. Since we humans are rebellious creatures, it never feels great to have things labeled as *forbidden*. Now that I'm recovered, this 90 percent philosophy is what I follow today. And by keeping a small margin of flexibility in my diet I feel like I'm getting the best of both worlds.

This chapter has been all about what to put in you — live probiotics and a whole-food plant-based diet. Yes, I did say that that means not eating animal products, but what I've tried to point out are critical foods that will truly fuel your recovery. Animal products will really throw a wrench in the system, and in my experience you should avoid them. And once you discover and start to enjoy the rainbow of plant-based deliciousness that's out there, I promise you you'll never look back.

8

TAKING A BREAK

Before CFS, it never would've occurred to me to *not eat* in an attempt to get well. When we are sick, whether we're hungry or not, we're so often told that we must eat in order to gain back our strength. Probably because humans evolved during times of scarcity, we seem to struggle to let go of that drive to eat as much as we can as often as we can. Although the fact that we evolved to thrive during times of scarcity probably also means that our bodies are used to (and probably rely on) getting a break from food once in a while.

Some of my biggest leaps forward with my health happened when I gave my body some breaks from solid food, and I'm confident that had I not incorporated some form of periodic fasting into my life, I never would've completely recovered from CFS.

Fasting, by definition, is the act of abstaining from all or some kinds of food or drink for a period of time. The kind of fasting that worked wonders for my CFS recovery (and the kind that I will be referring to every time I use this term from here on out) is any set period where you abstain from eating solid food. I'm not talking about going on a hunger strike like Gandhi — I allow myself healthy beverages such as water, freshly made vegetable juice, kombucha, or tea during a fast, but nothing else.

Although fasting eventually got easier, I cringe even just thinking about the day I attempted my first-ever fast. I imagine I probably boasted to others that I was doing the fast to improve my overall health, but this was a few years before I'd gotten sick with CFS, and truth be told, at that time I only really cared about losing weight. So with visions of my slimmed-down body in my head, I'd excitedly bought myself a shiny new juicer and stocked my fridge with enough vegetables to keep this fast of mine going for three full days.

I naively thought that it would be quite easy. I'd have fresh vegetable juice available to drink all day long, so really how bad could it be? I thought it would be like a laid-back little holiday of sorts where I didn't have to worry about cooking or lugging food around with me all day long. Surely it was going to be a breeze!

Getting through the first day of that bloody fast ended up feeling like one of the hardest things I'd ever had to do. I'd never before intentionally gone through a whole day without eating solid food, and that whole day I was obsessed with the fact that I wasn't eating. *How do I still have the energy to stand? Where am I getting my protein? I can't do this! I can't do this! I CAN'T DO THIS!*

My hunger felt intense and like almost more than I could bear. I white-knuckled it through that first day, but when I woke up on day two I was done. It was just too hard, and I didn't see how I could possibly get through the rest of day two, much less a third day. Honestly what it felt like to me was so much like torture. So with my juice cleanse officially abandoned I ended up tossing most of my vegetable stash in the trash because with this failed fast I'd also learned that eating that much produce in its whole form before it rots is virtually impossible. Feeling like a failure, I vowed that I'd never engage in this expensive, stressful, and ultimately wasteful experience ever again.

But once I had CFS, so much of what I read about healthy living insisted that fasting was an integral part of the healing process. It wasn't talked about as a diet, but instead as an efficient and effective pathway toward good health. For instance, in his book *The Blue Zones Solution*, Dan Buettner examines the regions of the world where people live the longest and shares the common practices that are found in each area that seem to be leading to this unusual longevity. Fasting, as it turns out (whether as a result of circumstance or choice), is a common occurrence among many of the world's healthiest and longest-lived communities.

As Buettner explains, fasting puts the cells in our bodies into an acute survival mode, which means cells produce fewer free radicals (the oxidizing agents that "rust" our bodies from the inside out). Lower levels of free radicals strengthen arteries, brain cells, and even the skin. Fasting also reduces levels of insulin-like growth factor 1 (IGF-1), a hormone important for cell growth in youth but potentially dangerous after about age twenty, as high levels may promote prostate, breast, and other cancers. His research also indicates that occasional fasting may stave off dementia by keeping blood vessels healthy and spurring brain cell growth. During fasting, cells also destroy viruses and harmful bacteria and get rid of damaged structures. It's a process, Buettner insists, that's critical for cell health, renewal, and survival.

The more I read on the topic, the more I knew there was no getting around my attempting another fast. But with this second go at fasting, having learned my lesson, I started small and bought only enough produce to last for a one-day fast. And what a relief it was when I discovered that this second attempt was much more manageable than my first attempt had been. It wasn't exactly *easy*, but it was *doable*. So with a newfound confidence in my fasting capabilities, I started experimenting with making these fasts a little bit longer.

My journey with fasting reminds me a bit of my journey with scuba diving. When I first started diving, I was really freaked out by the whole process. I found it terrifying being underwater without a natural air source nearby, and the first couple times I tried it I felt really panicky and scared. I couldn't think about anything other than getting my head back above water and couldn't figure out why anyone would possibly do this activity by choice. But by the end of my scuba certification course, being underwater and relying on a tank of compressed air barely bothered me at all. After a lifetime of associating being underwater with drowning, my mind simply needed some time to adjust to and trust this new way of breathing.

As with diving, when I first started fasting, my brain just needed some time to adjust to not eating and to trust that everything would be ok. At some point way back in the day I'm sure it was completely normal for humans to periodically go without food. But my spoiled body had never had to go without solid food for even one single day of its existence, so it took a bit of getting used to.

The beautiful thing about fasts is that you can use this time to do *nothing*. This is a time to simply relax and heal. Even now that I'm recovered and full of energy, when I fast I don't even have to find and decide to use that rarely used *off* switch of mine, because with the reduced calorie intake my body shifts me into low gear automatically. All that pressure I usually put on myself to be productive completely disappears. There are no chapters to write or sweaty workouts to complete. Those emails piling up in my inbox are not going to be touched. I'm not vacuuming or organizing cupboards or putting on makeup or polishing my toes. Fasting is the *only* thing on my schedule for the day. Fasting is something massive that I'm doing for my body, so all on its own it is enough. With my yoga pants on and hair in a ponytail, I curl up on the sofa with a green juice in one hand and a juicy novel that is teaching me *nothing* in the other and, with my hunger pangs forgotten, I get lost in the story.

These days, at some point, if I feel like it, I'll go for a walk. Not one of those brisk-counting-your-steps kinds of walks, but an honest-to-goodness stroll. One where I stop to smell and take pictures of the flowers. Where I sit back on the grass and gaze up at the beautiful cloud formations drifting above. If your current stage of illness and corresponding energy levels permit, in my experience this is also the perfect time for a massage. If you can afford it, book yourself in for an hour or two. If there's a healthy juice café nearby, stop by there afterward for a juicy tasty treat before you head home and finish off the day binge-watching your new favorite series. Peace, relaxation, and distraction — these are the keys to success while fasting.

Over the years I've experimented with different lengths of fasts, and I've concluded that three days is the maximum that my mind and body are comfortable doing. And many of my fasts aren't even this long. If I'm feeling at all under the weather, or feel I might have a touch of food poisoning, I'll do a quick twenty-four-hour fast just to help my body along. I find that the simple act of giving my body a full day to not have to deal with food allows it to heal much quicker than it would if I'd kept eating solid food.

<hr>

Although these periodic one- to three-day fasts helped me a lot, the biggest gains in my health came when I started incorporating **intermittent fasting** into my daily routine. By that I mean I'd give my body additional breaks from its food and digestion duties by *restricting* the number of hours during which I ate solid food each day. I found these smaller doses of fasting to be easier to do, and they proved to me that a little bit of something every day really can go a long way.

When suffering from CFS, I've found being gentle with our bodies is always key. Start small. Eat breakfast at 10:00 a.m. and dinner by 6:00 p.m. and see how that feels. Even with this modest fasting schedule you are still giving your body a sixteen-hour break from solid food. When you get used to this, shrink down your eating hours slightly. Try eating your first meal at 11:00 a.m. and your last one by 5:00 p.m. With just this simple habit you've now built in eighteen hours of fasting and healing time every single day.

Once the daily intermittent fasting has become routine, if you feel this is right for you, schedule for yourself a twenty-four-hour fast. After dinner on Monday night, don't eat again until dinner on Tuesday night. You can still have vegetable juice and kombucha and all the other healthy drinks out there; just don't eat any solid food between those two dinners. And boom — there you go! You've just successfully rocked your first twenty-four-hour fast.

Once the twenty-four-hour fasts feel manageable, push for longer once again. Ideally, you want to do a few of the longer fasts each year. I do four scheduled fasts each year lasting three days each. Set a regularly occurring reminder in your calendar that sends you a notification quarterly telling you that it's time to get juicing. And when that reminder pops up, eat dinner on Friday night and then don't eat solid food again until Monday's dinner. Over the weekend, illness and energy levels permitting, go visit some funky juice cafés and try to make the whole process a bit more enjoyable.

Remember that fasting isn't about not eating — it's about not eating solid food. That means if you're serious about fasting you're going to need to invest in a good quality juicer.

Think of this like dating. When picking out your juicer, if you don't choose something you want with you for the long haul, through good times and bad, you're going to have a rough go of things. Sure, in the juicer world there are some low-hanging-fruit types out there. They'll easily fit your budget, and you can grab one off the shelf and take it home today if you want to. They're fast and easy, but in the long run they are likely to disappoint. And in time, you'll see the shiny exterior start to break down. Eventually, when the honeymoon period wears off, you'll notice the flimsy construction and the fact that they half-ass it when juicing your produce. You'll need to buy twice as many vegetables to get half as much juice. That easy and cheap choice will end up costing you much more money and grief in the long run, and you'll wish you'd been more picky and done some more research and waited until you found The One before committing.

What you're looking for is a good quality cold-press juicer (or "masticating juicer"), as opposed to a centrifugal one. In contrast to the rough extraction and high speeds of centrifugal juicers, cold-press juicers operate at lower speeds and gently compress fruit and vegetables to "squeeze" out their juice. While more costly, their slower and more thorough extraction rates produce a higher-quality juice, and more of it.[1] With the cold-pressed option you'll be able to juice leafy greens, you'll get more juice out of everything you put in it, and your juice will last longer. These options are pricier and will run you in the US$300 – $700 range, but in the long run, they will prove their value many times over.

I have an Omega brand juicer that I've had for over a decade now that has worked great for me for every one of my fasts. I've lugged this heavy beast with me all over the world, and she has never once failed me. I've nicknamed her Earhart (after the first female pilot to fly solo across the Atlantic Ocean) because she's definitely no stranger to airplanes. She's been in backpacks and suitcases and had to adapt to all sorts of universal power and voltage settings, and she's always come through like a champ.

Let's talk about what to put into Zippy or whatever name you give to your juicer. The first step is to make up a big batch of vegetable juice each morning to keep in your fridge. Produce such as celery, cucumbers, bell peppers, zucchini, carrots, and beetroot work great. A good quality juicer will also juice healthy greens such as spinach, chard, kale, and parsley. You can add one apple, orange, or lemon for a touch of sweetness or acidity, which some people prefer, or add a bag of marshmallows if you want it sweeter.

I'm kidding about the marshmallows. But honestly, you can juice any fruit or vegetable you can imagine. When this all started I would have sworn that you wouldn't ever catch me combining kale and beets, or celery and lime, but now they're among my favorites.

Although the fasts definitely do get easier over time, I wouldn't go as far as to say that they're something that you will

look *forward* to. Despite them eventually feeling quite manageable, they still won't ever exactly be fun. But neither is washing
your car, or changing its oil, or scrubbing your toilets. I trust
that none of these are *ever* your first choice for how to spend
your day. But despite these things being a bit unpleasant, you
understand and appreciate that they need to be done. You care
about your car and your home, and so you take care of them.
And if you care about your body, you have to take care of it too.
A word to the wise: if you can, find a friend or ask your partner
or spouse to do it with you. Because just like scuba diving,
fasting is much more enjoyable and much less scary with a
buddy.

And don't feel you have to follow to the letter what any
books on the topic of fasting say (including this one!). In the
beginning, I was too strict with fasting and tried to follow too
closely the way other people did it, and as a result, I didn't
enjoy it and didn't want to do it very often. The reality is that
the only rules that exist for fasting are the ones you make.
Whatever you do, just find something that works for you so that
your body can start experiencing all the benefits that come with
this new awesomely healing habit of yours.

By now I *know* you're totally on board with eating and drinking
in ways that make you feel great. This has without question
become a no-brainer for you — the desire to be healthy and
happy and living the absolute best version of your life possible
is irresistible. Congratulations! This is amazing. Take a
moment, right here and now, and give yourself a hug. I mean it.
Wrap your arms around your body and declare to it out loud
that starting today you are going to treat it so well that it won't
know what to do with all the energy it's going to have.

So — now what? How do you pull all of this information together and, with what little energy you have, turn it all into a lifestyle change that will propel you toward your health goals?

The first thing that you need to understand - that you need to internalize and know from the depths of your soul — is that no one can lead you out of the CFS prison by changing your diet except for *you*.

Even your trusted doctor, as well-intentioned as he might be, likely can't help you out on this one. When I think back to my mother's time with CFS, I seriously doubt that anyone ever asked her about her diet. So much of the treatment she received from doctors was just symptom management. She was pre-scribed medication after medication after medication to help her better cope with the symptoms of CFS, but no one was ever trying to *cure* it. No one considered how what she put *in* her body might affect how that very body functioned.

Dr. Lim, the medical director at the TrueNorth Heath Centre, admits that, while completing his seven years of medical school, he didn't receive any training *at all* on food or on the impact that nutrition has on health. In preparing to become a doctor he didn't spend even one single hour learning about how food impacts health! It was only when Dr. Lim took it upon himself to learn about food's effect on the body that he came to understand the vital connection between the two. And during his time in medical school he was only taught how to *manage* chronic illness, but never taught how to reverse it. Over the years I've heard things like this before, but it never ceases to amaze me that this can possibly still be happening.

But as we've discussed, your doctor most likely can't be your one-stop-shop for answers. And that's perfectly ok, because in this Information Age, communication and informa-tion transmission are easier than ever. I encourage you to do your own research and find out more about the topics I just covered in the last two chapters.

I want to move on to talking about how to eat, but unfortunately, I need to stop and share some bad news. Unless you stop eating the "fantastically bad four" that I talk about in the next chapter, you'll really undo all the good you've done for yourself by eating probiotics, going WFPB, and fasting.

9

THE FANTASTICALLY BAD FOUR

While recovering from CFS (or any health issue for that matter), you obviously need to consume foods that help and support your body during the healing process. Eating too much of the wrong foods will keep you sick forever, and *nothing* is worth that price. Vibrant health is only possible with a vibrantly healthy diet — there's just no way around that. There unfortunately simply isn't any way to feel great while eating crap. Trust me, I've tried!

But I want to say that the crap isn't just crap. If only that was the worst of it! For those of us facing CFS, in my experience, these four items I'm about to get into here are practically toxic. It may sound overdramatic to say that, especially if you've never had CFS, but in truth, it's not. In fact, I think at some point in time we might look back on these four the way we look at cigarettes now.

There was a time when we were deceived by the health benefits of cigarettes. Some of us might be too young to have lived through this nonsense firsthand, but people were totally duped. Ads featured people actually doing physical activity while smoking, insisting that people looked chic and slender because they were smokers.

Eventually, the truth about smoking got out (that it leads to disease and disability and harms just about every organ system in the body), and slowly people started to wise up.[1] Sure, that first puff might smell pretty good, but after a while cigarettes smell pretty gross, and I don't find a hacking cough all that attractive myself. Once a disturbing picture of some diseased body part was slapped on the package (that's what they do in Canada) along with a warning saying something like *smoking kills*, many of us began to accept that this cherished habit was likely the end of us, and that we needed to somehow find a way to quit.

Well, I'm about to say the same about some cherished food habits. Whether we're actually addicted to them or not is not the issue. The simple fact is that we go through our lives talking, acting, and yes, even thinking that we need these things the same way someone who is addicted to cigarettes talks, acts, and even thinks about their next cigarette. That's the opposite of being free, folks, and if there's one thing I could give all my readers, it would be freedom from CFS. As far as I'm concerned, eating these four things is the equivalent of putting the shackles on yourself.

In the past, my drug of choice was definitely **sugar**, and I really hate to think about all the damage that all this sugar consumption was doing to my body. No joke - I was one of those *over the top, binge eating, had to get my fix on the regular* types. When I gave in to my cravings (which happened A LOT), whatever convenience store or bakery I hit up would have to order more stock once I left. I knew it was bad for me, but for the longest time, I just couldn't stop. I tried over and over, through willpower alone, to cut back on sugary foods. It never worked. This felt bigger than me, like no matter how hard I tried or how badly I wanted to quit, there was just no way it was possible. There was a sugar-loving beast inside of me who demanded she get her fix, and she was much too big to tame. Plus, sugar was a total happiness elixir for me, and I couldn't imagine living a life without it.

I was certain it was just my weak will power, but it turns out that there was something physiological happening that at the time I didn't at all understand. I now know that eating foods containing added sugar (that is, sugar not occurring naturally in food) gives your brain a surge of a feel-good chemical called dopamine, and it also raises your blood sugar levels fast giving you an immediate burst of energy. And then, as fast as all this happens, it all slips away, leaving you feeling jittery, anxious, depressed, exhausted, and once again craving more sugar.[2]

And if only that dreaded sugar crash were the worst of your problems. According to Dr. Robert Lustig, an endocrinologist and medical professor at the University of California, added sugar should be thought of in the exact same way as cigarettes or alcohol — as something that's killing us.[3] He insists it's not about the calories — it's that sugar itself is a poison likely responsible for much of the heart disease, hypertension, common cancers, and many other chronic ailments we see today. The Mayo Clinic reports that poor nutrition, weight gain, increased triglycerides, and tooth decay also result from added sugar.[4] Sugar also increases inflammation and joint pain and causes liver, pancreas, kidney, and skin damage.

Unfortunately, I know it's not just me. As a culture, we've been duped about sugar. Most poisons come with warning labels, but our culture views sugar as one of life's most precious gifts. Whether it's household cleaners or cigarettes, we know just by looking at the packaging that they are going to harm us if we consume them. Baked goods and other sugary treats, on the other hand, are packaged up beautifully. They're colorful and pretty and their appearance brings us joy even before we've started eating them. Cakes remind us of treasured childhood birthday parties and of going to fun-filled weddings with family and friends. Chocolate reminds us of Easter and of heart-shaped gifts received from the people we love. But underneath the pretty package is a dopamine trigger system that will completely undo all the hard work you've put in up to this point.

If you currently consume added sugar in your diet, just by reading books like this one and understanding the harmful effects of added sugar, you're already on your way to putting this health-destroying habit behind you. I've found that once you shine a bright light on a bad habit, the denial disappears pretty quickly. The next step is to load yourself up with fermented foods. I've truly found this to be a game changer. This way your microbiome won't be contributing to your cravings, and you will be ready to kick this sugar habit for good.

And the great news is that will power has nothing to do with this process. We'll get into this in much more detail in chapters 17 and 18, but for now know that true behavior change is all about information, awareness, planning, and skills. It's something that can be learned and implemented by virtually anyone. Once you understand how to develop new habits and shape your environment in a way that supports healthy choices, you'll be putting this bad habit behind you for good.

For a long time, **alcohol** was another tricky one for me to get under control. Like sugar, alcohol also at times felt too big and strong of a force to try to master. On countless occasions "a couple of drinks" has turned into WAY more than planned, and no matter how many times I swore it'd be the last, I seemed doomed to keep repeating this same behavior. It was another struggle that I'd assumed I'd have to endure for life.

And then I found a gem of a book called *This Naked Mind: Control Alcohol, Find Freedom, Discover Happiness, & Change Your Life*, in which author Annie Grace points a vital spotlight at just how destructive to our health alcohol consumption can be. Truthfully, I'd mostly thought of my overindulgence with alcohol as more of an embarrassing social habit than as something that was actually killing me. But Grace explains in detail how clever advertising campaigns have glorified alcohol consumption to the point that we don't even see it as a toxic drug anymore. There is so much manipulation that goes on behind the scenes to get us to this place where most of us don't even see how horrible this drug habit of ours really is. We've been convinced that quitting or seriously restricting our alcohol intake is too hard to even try and that not drinking will, without a doubt, be a form of social suicide.

I have found that alcohol consumption and CFS recovery absolutely do not mix. Not even a little bit. When you drink, even though you're unable to see the damage that alcohol does to your internal organs, it's definitely happening. It weakens your heart, changes your brain structure, damages your pancreas, causes potentially life-threatening liver damage, and leads to heart disease, diabetes, and cancer.[5]

I'll admit, this alcohol abstinence was a tough one for me to come to terms with because there were times during my CFS journey when consuming alcohol felt on par with suddenly having a superpower. During my earliest days with CFS when I could barely get out of bed I doubt that pounding back a couple of cocktails would have had any sort of positive effect, but during those later years when I existed in a sort of half sick, half recovered state, alcohol could make me feel almost "normal" again. A sloppy, slurring, tripping over myself normal, but *normal* nonetheless. Normal enough to last through a dinner party and keep up with my peers. Normal enough to have energy and completely forget about the concept of naps. Normal enough to feel, at least for a few hours, like I was actually living again.

I wish I could tell you what was happening in my body when I consumed alcohol with CFS, but the truth is I have no clue. In my experience it's all very mysterious, alluring, and dangerous. The high of intoxication might have temporarily allowed me to move through life as if CFS didn't exist, but the hangovers would level me. And in time I came to see that without a doubt my alcohol consumption and abuse kept me frozen in CFS amber, unable to heal until I put the bottle down.

In their book *Undo It! How Simple Lifestyle Changes Can Reverse Most Chronic Diseases*, Dr. Dean Ornish and Anne Ornish explain that consuming even just one alcoholic drink per day increases your risks for certain types of cancer; the largest study ever done on the health effects of alcohol consumption in 195 countries concluded that the widely held views of the health benefits of alcohol need revising. This study exposed flaws in the previous research making claims that alcohol could improve health and revealed that there is, in fact, no safe limit. That despite this being in conflict with most healthy drinking guidelines, the safest level of drinking is actually none.

If alcohol use is something that is an issue for you, it's time to take action. Schedule for yourself a complete break from alcohol, even if just for a couple weeks. Once you get a couple weeks under your belt, try committing to a month, then even longer. In *This Naked Mind*, Grace teaches us that when we take breaks from alcohol we can interrupt our habits and take back control. So set up your environment to support your sobriety. Remove alcohol from your home and meet friends for coffee instead of drinks. Little by little you'll start to see that you are so much happier and healthier without booze.

When you are in the throes of CFS, **caffeine** also has to go. Now I know that for many people this is an unthinkable statement that I just made, but hear me out. When I was at my worst with this illness, caffeine always did me more harm than good. With CFS, caffeine is an energy loan shark, always taking much more than it gives.

Doctors overwhelmingly advise against caffeine intake when you have CFS.[6] Dr. Jacob Teitelbaum, medical director of the national Fibromyalgia and Fatigue Centers warns caffeine aggravates adrenal exhaustion and low blood sugars, amplifying anxiety, stress symptoms, and fatigue.

When you are chronically low on energy, I know it can be incredibly tempting to consume something that will give you a boost for a while. All I'm asking is that you be aware of how your body reacts to it, and be mindful of what the ultimate cost of this little boost is in the end. While sick, caffeine will put you on a stressful energy rollercoaster. Sure, you'll get a nice little pick-me-up for a while, but the inevitable crash that follows will be intense. Once I removed caffeine I found that some of the afternoon fatigue that I was attributing to CFS was actually just my caffeine crash. With CFS your energy levels are in such a fragile state that messing around with caffeine is something that you just cannot afford to do.

So how do you just ditch this liquid that has become as

much of a life force in your day as air or water? I found that slowly weaning myself off first was key, and then finding an enjoyable replacement to take its place totally did the trick for me. Now for all you coffee snobs, you're probably not going to love this plan but what I found worked best was to make my coffee at home using *instant coffee* (it's really so much better than it sounds) and slowly lower the caffeine content with each passing day. You can accomplish this by buying a jar of both caffeinated and decaffeinated instant coffee and then use a mix of both when you make your cup for the morning. As time goes on, slowly add in more decaffeinated and less caffeinated until you are drinking completely decaf coffee. Because don't you find that much of the enjoyment from coffee comes from the ritual? From here, you can stick with the decaf, or else switch it for something else like green tea or kombucha because again, just having a cup of *something* to enjoy is usually enough to keep us happy.

Once your health starts to improve, I've found that you can slowly start consuming some caffeine again (if you like), but only ever in small quantities. When it comes to people with CFS or a history of CFS, I firmly believe that they always need to be extremely careful with their caffeine intake. I suspect that even when the healthiest of people throw high doses of caffeine into their bodies it's not doing them any good.

Once you are feeling strong enough and recovered enough to start having some caffeine again, take measures to control how much you're consuming. When you make coffee at home use one-third regular and two-thirds decaf so that the caffeine content isn't too high. When you buy your iced Americanos (or lattes or cappuccinos or whatever) in coffee shops, regardless of what size you order, always ask the barista to only put one shot of espresso in it. Or use half decaf. Or make it half water. Or better yet, order green tea! Your healthy energized body won't need the high doses of caffeine to feel good anyway, so there's no reason to risk taxing your system needlessly.

When I look at the people in life who I want to be like — the ones who are healthy and strong and just generally awesome — when I see them in the food court or at a buffet, I look at what's on their plate. I see what lines they are standing in. I can tell you that they are almost never in line at the pizza or waffle place and that their plates are usually filled with health-promoting whole foods. There's not a potato chip in sight. Indeed, despite the diversity of foods that healthy people eat, if there's one thing in common it's that they don't eat **processed foods**.

What do I mean by processed foods? These are foods that don't really resemble anything that comes from nature. Processed foods, as they are, can't be grown or picked or peeled. Think of things like breakfast cereals, candy bars, cakes, crackers, ramen noodles, and soft drinks. Basically everything you can buy at a gas station. But it doesn't stop there. Those "healthy" and "lean" ready-made meals in the frozen foods aisle at your local organic grocery store often fall into this category too. Even vegetables — if they come in cans — are culprits here. Deli meats, sausages, and bacon are all highly processed. Many household staples such as ketchup, margarine, and granola bars fall into this category also. Typically anything that has a label or comes in a can or box should probably be avoided as fuel for a body recovering from CFS.

Processed foods cause a lot of problems, first and foremost being that they are *so* easy to overeat. Dr. Garth Davis, a weight loss surgeon at The Davis Clinic who's also interviewed in *What the Health*, explains how obesity is a death sentence that puts you at a much higher risk for getting a whole host of diseases. He points out how this movement to make us comfortable with our overweight bodies, as well-intentioned as it might be, is making us comfortable with being sick. Our bodies simply do not thrive when in this condition, and just about every disease he sees is because of what people are eating.

We think junk food is what makes life enjoyable, don't we? But a life spent enslaved by food addictions is no life at all. Television shows and movies can be especially bad for giving people the impression that you can eat and drink all the junk you want and still look and feel great. We forever see healthy and fit people on TV whose characters are drinking alcohol every day and eating tons of junk food, and that is just not reality. The people who actually eat and drink toxic junk every day are sick and overweight, and they look terrible.

And when it comes to your food, keep it simple. Forget all the complex *loophole* meals and snacks like "chicken fingers" made out of tofu and rolled in corn flakes, dipped in a sauce of stevia and corn starch. This stuff is expensive and time-consuming to make and is never as satisfying as you think it will be (and probably not all that healthy). When I first started to really turn my diet around, I put a lot of effort into trying to somehow replace all the junk food I was used to eating with healthy versions of it. But the replacement cheat foods never really tasted that good and were so exhausting to make. And for most junk food there really just isn't a healthy version to swap with. Learn from me and don't even bother with this. Get into the habit of eating real food, and before you know it you won't miss the junk or feel the need to replicate it one bit. In time, you'll find that you don't even care so much about that "treat" anymore.

Once I finally left the junk food behind for good, I realized that I enjoyed my weekends (the time during which I usually had my *treats*) more when I ate healthy food. Once you start to notice how much better you feel when you eat well, dealing with the after-effects of that massive weekend brunch will no longer seem worth it. And after having eaten healthy food consistently for a while, the crappy food out there will lose much of its appeal. So ditch the crap, because it's time to get on the same team as your body and get well.

Does this mean that I've removed every single harmful thing and bad habit from my life? No, it doesn't. But I have committed to ditching the Fantastically Bad Four, and I can tell you that if you start there, it makes life so much easier. What it means is that, as time goes by, I eliminate more and more of the bad stuff and replace it with more and more of the good. I doubt I'll ever achieve perfection in this area, but I'm definitely aiming for something close to it. Now that I've gotten my microbiome in order, green meal planning in place, and built up some great habits, it's easier to stay away from foods that are literally imprisoning my body.

Now that you know what to eat (and what not to eat) to get well, in the next chapter I'm going to talk more about *how* to eat to get well.

10

MAKING FOOD WORK FOR YOU

It's a great start to know what to eat and what not to eat, but *how* you eat turns out to be just as important. And you might be wondering, how strict do I have to be with all of this? How much commitment to this new way of eating is necessary?

We like to say that everything is ok in moderation, but I don't think that's true. Dr. Patrick Flynn, author of *I Disagree: How These Two Words are the Secret to Thinking Differently and Taking Control of Your Health* insists that moderation is the word we use to justify our toxic eating habits. If something is poisoning your body, it's poisonous no matter what quantity you consume it in. And it's not like the food industry believes in moderation. They want you to finish whatever you're eating so you'll buy another. They're not even hiding that fact ("Bet you can't eat just one!").

Don't be fooled by the childish voice in your head that tells you dozens of reasons why consuming unhealthy food and drinks isn't harmful to you. You have to be your own parent here and keep yourself in line because, as an adult, no one else will. Listen to the grownup voice in your head, the one that reminds you of what's important and what's true.

I frequently hear sentiments like *life is too short to skip dessert*. I say, life is too short *unless* you skip dessert! Life is too short not to take care of yourself. Life is too short not to treasure your body and treat it with the respect it deserves. Life is too short not to make sure you're living the healthiest, happiest version possible.

And when we allow ourselves small quantities of a food that we struggle with, life can become all about getting to that one moment when we get to have it. You are still a slave to that food, and indulging in it can be a gateway to chaos and to a giant leap backward. When you completely remove the items in your diet that you battle with the most, it can be incredibly freeing and make your life so much easier.

You can see what I mean if you think about this in the context of cigarettes. It's really nonsense to suggest that you can smoke cigarettes in moderation. They're addictive! Sure there's always that one outlier that claims they have one every now and then without issue, but the other 99% of us get hooked big time. The whole point is that they want you to finish that pack so you have to buy another. Cigarettes are designed to allow you to cave in to your cravings like a little kid — to justify smoking one because "life is too short" to deny yourself the pleasure of lung cancer. And a life of moderation with cigarettes is a life spent waiting for your next cigarette. It's not a life free of cigarettes — it's a life dictated by cigarettes.

Now think about the same thing with an apple. You're never, ever going to find yourself saying "I should really eat this apple in moderation." No one (most of all yourself) would think badly of you for "caving" in to your cravings for a crisp sweet apple. And come to think of it, healthy kids really do crave apples! Does anyone eating an apple ever have to justify it by saying, "Life is too short not to eat this apple?" And I don't see anyone looking at the clock waiting for the next chance they can get to eat an apple. There's no designated apple-eating area and no one furtively eats one either. You can just see the absurdity of even trying to imagine these things with an apple. And that's precisely my point. Food should feel like nourishment, not a drug.

I'm sure there's one thing on the Fantastically Bad Four list that's really going to be a sacrifice for you. Let's say it's alcohol. Am I saying that you're *never* allowed to drink again?

First off, you're *allowed* to drink whenever you want. YOU are the boss. Always. You just need to be mindful of the cost and decide if that tasty little buzz is worth heading back to CFS jail. Once you've *recovered* from CFS it's probably ok to drink on occasion, but when you do, always have a plan. During my old irresponsible drinking days, I'd head out for the night, keep a drink in hand from start to finish and just cross my fingers that as the night went on I might somehow miraculously make smart decisions regarding my alcohol consumption. And as I'm sure you've already guessed (or know from experience), that never works.

But that's *once* you've recovered. When you're trying to get better, you have to honestly ask yourself: is a drink worth the setback? After consuming alcohol, research shows that many CFS sufferers experience increased tiredness, increased nausea, exacerbated hangovers, and sleep disturbance.[1] Essentially, one of the many *gifts* of CFS is that if you drink, even in small quantities, you almost certainly have a Super Hangover waiting for you every single time. And with CFS you basically feel like you *already* have a hangover all the time, even without drinking. So why on earth would you ever want to add to your already considerable suffering?

In a nutshell, what I'm saying is that it's time to get all your addictions under control. I'm willing to bet that there's at least one toxic thing in your life that at times feels bigger and stronger than you. Maybe it's sugar or greasy fatty foods or nicotine or other harmful drugs. Whatever it is, just be honest about the damage these things are causing and the extent to which they're keeping you from reaching your goals.

If you feel like you must have a drink (or eat some sugar, or eat a bag of chips, etc.), I think you should plan for it. If you decide that you want to have a couple drinks every now and then, look at your calendar and pick no more than one weekend per month when you will consume alcohol. And then on that scheduled night, before you take even one sip of your first drink, state out loud to someone else (who you trust will be drinking responsibly) how many drinks you will have over the course of the night. By sharing your plan with someone else, you have accountability to stick to your plan. Then, mentally plan out the timing (one at dinner, two at the party afterward). On top of that, alternate your alcoholic drinks with water (or alternate a bag of chips with an apple, etc.).

Or stick to not drinking at all. Try keeping a sparkling water with lime in hand and just let others assume it's alcohol. I've found that when I'm at any social event, as long as I have liquid of some kind in my hand (alcoholic or otherwise), I'm completely content. If your illness has you stuck at home - stock your fridge with a case of kombucha instead of a box of wine. If you love to snack, then snack on apple slices. If caffeine is your thing, then how about a no-sugar-added fruit juice? But whatever you do, make sure you completely avoid those specific situations that you know will be an issue for you. If night clubs or free-flow happy hour specials more often than not end up getting messy, stop going to these places. If curling up on the couch leads to sugar binges, then don't. Sit up in a chair, or better yet, (health permitting) go for a walk.

It's amazing how once our bodies and minds adjust to not indulging in bad eating habits, we find comfort and joy in new, healthier things. I used to love smoking, but I can't imagine ever feeling joy or comfort from a cigarette ever again. Instead, now I get an insane amount of pleasure from eating a bowl of cherries while sipping on some apple green tea kombucha. Homemade granola is now in the *to die for* category. And don't even get me started on garlic and artichoke hummus! In short, trust the process, give it time, and all the "sacrifices" (giving up cleverly disguised poisons) soon won't feel like sacrifices at all.

There are no boxes of cookies or bags of potato chips in my pantry. There are no more booze-fueled benders that end when the sun comes up. And for someone trying to recover from CFS, snacking on sugar and powering through your day on caffeine is the same as smoking cigarettes. I certainly don't feel deprived or that it takes any discipline or willpower to keep this up. In reality, my life is actually so much better and easier not having any sort of food battles or willpower decisions to make when it comes to my eating and drinking. I have a plan, and I stick to it. That's it.

And that's where I want to go next — to having a plan. Once you know what foods promote healing and which ones don't, there are so many things that you can do to set yourself up to be successful with a healthy eating plan that will ensure you stay on track. None of this has to be hard or unpleasant or frustrating — if you have a plan. When it comes to eating food, always have a plan. Did I mention that you should have a plan?! Having a plan takes out all the guesswork and ensures your weeks run smoothly.

If you're well enough to manage your own meal planning, set a weekly reminder for this on your calendar, and when it pops up sit down and make a plan for what you'll eat the following week. I use a really simple planning chart that I made myself and keep in a handy place on my computer. It has seven columns across the top, one for each day of the week, and four columns down the side, one each for breakfast, lunch, snack, and dinner.

Whatever type of planning chart you use, use the same template each week, and make sure every single thing that you're going to eat or drink the following week goes on that chart. Some of the items that you consume each week repeatedly can stay on the template. (List them in bold or highlight them so you remember to keep them there.) The rest you can fill in week-by-week as you go.

When CFS is at its worst I know that your meals will need to stay simple, because the energy required for masterful culinary creations unfortunately just isn't there. Toss some veggies on a baking sheet and throw them in the oven. Serve that up with a piece of wholegrain sourdough bread and a handful of nuts (or whatever healthy foods agree with you). Despite your meals not being all that exciting, they will give your body what it needs to heal, and that is most important. If you're not up to doing your own meal planning, make sure that the person or service in charge of your meals knows the deal. The point is (as I might have mentioned) - there always needs to be a plan!

Once your health starts to improve, you'll regain the luxury of getting to be a bit more creative. Now it's time to set the Pinterest website as the homepage on your computer browser so that every single time you want to find something on the Internet, this is the first page that you'll see. Pinterest is great in that every time you open it you get a fresh page of suggestions for you based on your past searches within the site. Let's say you've already clicked on a few recipes for salads, soups, and other healthy dishes. With Pinterest as your homepage, each time you open your browser, it will bring up new healthy options for you to peruse.

What I do is each time I open the browser on my computer, I take thirty seconds to look at the list of suggestions there waiting for me on my Pinterest homepage. When I see a tasty meal option I want to try, I click on it and add it to one of my Pinterest boards (files you create to keep your items organized). I recommend you keep separate boards for vegetables, soups, salads, grains, and so on.

By committing to taking thirty seconds each time you open your browser to look at what recipes are suggested and saving the ones you like, in a bunch of small doses, you quickly and easily build up an excellent personalized collection of great recipes. Or if this still seems like more than you can manage at the moment, just use the Pinterest board of recipes I've collected. Visit https://www.pinterest.ca/raelanagle/ and you can make use of my ever-growing collection of healthy and delicious meal ideas.

When making your meal plan for the week, pick a recipe you want to try from one of your (or my) Pinterest boards, and note its name on your meal planning chart in the time slot where you plan to make it (for example: *Monday – Dinner*). Then take a screenshot of the recipe and put the screenshot into the folder on your computer where your meal planning chart is stored. If you don't want to save a screenshot of the recipe, you can instead just pull up the recipe on Pinterest when you need to get the ingredients and make the dish. Or print it out if that works better for you.

On your meal planning chart also add in any snacks you

plan to have, as well as all the beverages you will consume. If you start each day with a glass of fresh lemon water, that goes on the chart. If you regularly drink kombucha or other teas, then they go on the chart as well. If you leave something off the chart, it's almost guaranteed that you'll forget to buy what you need for it. When you put absolutely everything you consume on the chart, it becomes much easier to figure out what ingredients and supplies you'll need to buy to be ready for the week to come.

To get you started, I'm sharing a week's worth of my favorite recipes already organized in a meal planning chart with the recurring items indicated in bold. My meals are usually a bit more repetitive than this, but I mixed it up a bit here so that you can get a glimpse at what some more options could look like. You certainly don't need to commit to making all of these, but if you're up to the task it certainly would be a tasty week! You can find all the recipes for the meals listed by visiting https://www.pinterest.ca/raelanagle/raelans-one-week-meal-plan/.

MEAL PLAN	MONDAY	TUESDAY	WEDNESDAY	THURSDAY	FRIDAY	SATURDAY	SUNDAY
BREAKFAST	Spinach & Mango Smoothie Bowl	Spinach & Mango Smoothie Bowl	Spinach & Mango Smoothie Bowl	Blueberry Muffin Smoothie Bowl	Blueberry Muffin Smoothie Bowl	Amazing Tofu Scramble	
LUNCH	Cilantro Avocado White bean Dip; Carrot Sticks; Toasted Wholewheat Sourdough; Sauerkraut	Cilantro Avocado White bean Dip; Carrot Sticks; Toasted Wholewheat Sourdough; Sauerkraut	Cilantro Avocado White bean Dip; Carrot Sticks; Toasted Wholewheat Sourdough; Sauerkraut	Vegan Green Goddess Pasta Salad; Sauerkraut	Vegan Green Goddess Pasta Salad; Sauerkraut	Vegan Green Goddess Pasta Salad; Sauerkraut	Brunch Out
SNACK	Kombucha; Bowl of Mixed Berries	Kombucha; Bowl of Mixed Berries	Kombucha; Bowl of Mixed Berries	Kombucha; Mixed Nuts & Chopped Raw Veggies	Kombucha; Mixed Nuts & Chopped Raw Veggies	Kombucha; Mixed Nuts & Chopped Raw Veggies	Kombucha; Mixed Nuts & Chopped Raw Veggies
DINNER	One Pot Quinoa	One Pot Quinoa	One Pot Quinoa	Roasted Cauliflower Bowl with Tahini Dressing	Roasted Cauliflower Bowl with Tahini Dressing	Dinner Out / Order In	Red Lentil & Spinach Masala

After you've got your meal plan for the week all filled out, you then need to figure out what you need to buy to make everything. Your best bet at efficiency in this department is going to be using a mobile app. I know most of us are still rocking that unorganized little piece of paper with items messily scribbled on it, but there really is such a better way to do this.

For my grocery list I use an app called Anylist. I've tried a bunch of different ones over the years, and by far I've found this one to be the best for groceries. It's free, it's easy to use, and it organizes my lists just how I like them. I prefer to find free ways to do things, but if you choose to pay for the pro version of Anylist you can even do your meal planning and collect your recipes in this app too.

You definitely don't have to master everything all at once. Start small and over time slowly work your way up to your end goal of where you want to be with food, because no one gets everything perfect on Day One.

To figure out what needs to go on the list, first open up your meal planning chart. Start at the beginning of the week with the first meal (the top left corner of the chart), and one by one go through each item listed until you've covered them all. Look at the screenshots of your chosen recipes (or grab your printouts or open up the recipes on Pinterest), and go through the ingredient lists to see what you need and add those items to your app. Anylist automatically organizes everything into categories such as *produce* and *frozen foods,* so it's easy for you when you get to the grocery store to stay organized and get what you need.

You can also create a separate list for each of the main

grocery stores you usually go to, and then as you need items that you know you can only get at a specific store you can add them to that list. I try to rotate the grocery stores I visit and only hit one each week and stock up on the items I need from each one while I'm there. If you're not up fo grocery shopping, many cities have reasonably priced grocery delivery services available for use. There are many apps out for this these days and a quick Google search will tell you which ones will work best for you where you live.

And a final word of advice about grocery shopping: don't *ever* buy a single thing at the grocery store that isn't on your list. Since your home is a junk-free zone and you already have a plan for all the food you will eat the next week, there is never a reason to deviate from your list. Stick to the plan to give yourself the best shot at being healthy.

Since processed food is not on your shopping list, health permitting — you're going to find yourself in the kitchen cooking. I find making healthy homemade food really therapeutic. It took some time to get to that point, but now I truly appreciate how amazing it is to have the energy and the means to prepare fresh and healthy food every single day. It's a privilege that unfortunately far too many people do not get to enjoy. When I look at all the beautiful ingredients I'm using, I get really excited about how nourishing this food will be for my body. I think about all the healing properties these ingredients have and how much this food will help me to achieve my health and fitness goals.

If you're up for it, to get ready for the week, wash and air dry all the produce you'll need for the week on Monday so that it's ready to go when you need it (or suggest to the cook in your home that they do this). To keep your life simple, try eating the same thing for breakfast every day. If you do this for lunch as well, this practice will really save you time and energy. If there is any meal prep necessary for either breakfast or lunch (such as chopping vegetables or cooking up a batch of quinoa), prep that all at the beginning of the week so that you have the containers of food ready to go for the rest of the week. I find it's much easier to prep a big batch all at once than to get small batches ready to eat every single day.

For dinner, try sticking to only two different meals for the week: one that you'll eat Monday to Wednesday, and another that you'll eat Thursday and Friday. This adds a bit more variety into your diet, but it isn't so complicated that you have to worry about preparing something new every single evening. On weekends, give yourself a break from cooking and order in (something healthy). Or if you're feeling up to it, go check out some organic cafés or vegan restaurants in your neighborhood. Or keep cooking! Whatever floats your boat. With a healthy diet food still can and will be an enjoyable part of your life. Make foods that inspire you. Visit cafés that energize you. Whatever you do, make it fun!

I've just bombarded you with several chapters of information about food, but I want to leave you with a final piece of advice. I don't know who's responsible for it, but one of my favorite sayings is *Don't let the perfect be the enemy of the good*. Essentially, be dedicated to healthy eating, but don't beat yourself up on the occasions you happen to fall short. If you slip up, don't use that one minor error in judgment as an excuse to make a dozen more unhealthy decisions with your diet. Don't fall apart because there was an open bag of potato chips at a party and you had a handful, or you went out for ice cream because you just moved to a new city and a friend raved about the ice cream there.

With that said, as much as possible, always make healthy eating a priority, because I'm confident that so much of your success will be determined by what is on your plate. So much of your happiness will come from getting over your food addictions. It can be a bit of work to get your diet on track, but the payoff when you break out of the CFS prison will be huge. Once you do it, you'll wonder why you didn't do it sooner. It's such a game-changer and, in the end, feels like a no-brainer. Put in some effort and get the right things on your plate, and your future self will definitely thank you for it.

V

FREE TO MOVE

11

UNDERSTANDING YOUR EXERCISE PATH

When we're tired, we rest. It's that simple. Isn't it? If we're especially tired, we rest even more. Right? For most of us, the antidote to exhaustion is and always has been sleep. Even if we're not experts at listening to our bodies, most of us know how to figure out at least this much.

When CFS first hit me, I'd been running myself into the ground for most of my adult life. With the perpetual sleep debt I carried around, it wasn't surprising when my body finally started to protest. I assumed that my feelings of extreme fatigue were my body's way of forcing me to slow down and finally get some much-needed rest and recovery time.

I knew that this was a complicated illness and that there were likely other parts to the recovery equation, but regardless of what else I was going to have to do to get well, I was certain that rest was going to be a big part of the process.

So for quite a while, I did just that. I devoured books and binge-watched TV series and basically did anything I could think of that would keep me entertained while glued to my bed or couch. I simplified my days, minimized my obligations, and cut back on my chores, all in an effort to ensure that I'd spend as many hours as possible resting up.

The weeks and months went by and, much to my astonishment and frustration, all this rest wasn't getting me *one iota better*. No matter how much rest I got, I was still completely exhausted and sick. It was baffling. This beast known as CFS was some kind of monster that I clearly did not understand, one that relentlessly dragged me down and couldn't be stopped by conventional methods.

One thing that did become clear was that I was not going to be able to *rest* my way out of this.

———

There was something that I was missing, something that I wasn't grasping about this illness, and I knew I needed to find another approach to healing if I wanted to get well. Dr. M. had always stressed that exercise would be an important part of my recovery from CFS. Since for a long time I'd loved to exercise, I assumed that this part of my healing plan would be a piece of cake.

I know that there are a lot of people who need significant motivation to work out, and it's a struggle for them to get to the gym. And at one point in time, that definitely used to be me. But thankfully, as time passed, that was no longer the case. It seems all that time spent during my twenties dragging myself to the gym slowly rewired those reward centers in my brain to crave exercise, and eventually, I got to a point where my body was flooded with dopamine every time I hit the gym. In fact, when it came to exercise, by the time I got sick my issues with self-control were around keeping myself from doing *too much*.

But attempting to work out with CFS felt like trying to exercise with a bad flu. It felt like I was walking through wet concrete — concrete that beat me up once I got through it. Despite feeling so incredibly ill, when I first got sick I tried doing some really light exercises at home, but it just felt impossible. No matter how *little* I did, I always felt so much worse afterward. Although still a struggle, my days without exercise could be bearable. With exercise, life felt impossible. So eventually I just stopped trying. I got angry at exercise, and for a while I convinced myself that with CFS exercise would only ever serve to make me worse. And if anyone even so much as *hinted* that I should try exercising to get better, they would get an earful from me on why that was a terrible idea.

My inability to exercise might just have been the hardest thing with which I had to come to terms with with CFS. I never got used to it, and I was never able to fully accept it. I raged against my inability to be physically active for my entire decade with this illness. I wanted to exercise so badly, but I just couldn't. And there were so many able-bodied people out there that could exercise but just couldn't be bothered to, and the injustice of it all made me livid. My mind was there and completely on board with the idea. I was ready to shred some crazy-ass workouts. But my body just wouldn't cooperate.

I fantasized all the time about being able to return to the gym. Because I missed it so incredibly much, every now and then I'd put my anger and frustration with my past failed attempts aside and give exercise another try. *Maybe this time it won't be that bad. Maybe this time I'll find the magic formula that will make it all possible.*

But no matter what I tried, or how light of an activity it was, that small amount of exercise always left me feeling terrible. Every single time. There was always a steep price to pay for my efforts. A price that was often more than I could afford while trying to keep up with the demands of the rest of my life. I already felt like I was getting through life by the skin of my teeth and just barely keeping up with whatever commitments I had. When I attempted to add any form of physical activity to my life, keeping up with everything else felt impossible. Exercise felt like a one-way trip back to the slammer.

There just seemed to be no way to manage all the pain and downtime that came with experimenting with an exercise program while I had to keep up with so many other demands and responsibilities. Even if the actual exercise itself only took up a couple minutes of my day, the recovery time could wipe out the rest of it, and possibly days afterward too. Before I could bring exercise into my life effectively, I was sure something else significant had to give, and for quite a few years, I just didn't make this critical aspect of healing enough of a priority to ever be successful with it. For a long time, it never felt like I could possibly give anything up to make that space for an exercise program. I was stuck in the moment and figuring out how to survive each day instead of focusing on the big picture and figuring out how I was going to survive the rest of my life.

In spite of my struggles with exercise, deep down I maintained the belief that physical activity would eventually be an integral part of my getting well. This was something that just made good intuitive sense to me. I'd also seen this in action to a small degree during my time scuba diving when small doses of exertion actually started making me feel a bit stronger. It was always there in the back of my mind as something I would start once my life allowed for it — once my responsibilities were fewer and I had the space in my life for all the sick days that past experience had shown me exercise would bring.

It wasn't just my *gut* telling me to get active — experts also drove home the reality that exercise needs to happen for our bodies to heal and thrive. In their book *Younger Next Year: Live Strong, Fit, and Sexy — Until You're 80 and Beyond*, Chris Crowley and Henry S. Lodge, MD, explain the importance of doing something physical each and every day so that your body gets the signals it needs telling it that it's time to thrive. Exercise triggers waves of "grow" messages throughout your body. When you get your body moving, you create a surge that changes the activity and biology of virtually every organ and muscle in your body.

Being sedentary, on the other hand, is the most important signal to your body that it's time to decay. In the environment that our bodies evolved to thrive, there was no reason to be sedentary except famine. Your body watches what you do, and that lack of physical activity sends the message that it's time to *die*. Regardless of how much food you eat, that's what you tell your body every day that you *don't* exercise.

So when that beautiful window of opportunity opened up for me, I knew I finally had my chance to try to get active again. Once I'd quit my job and had the support of a loving partner, at last I had the time and space I needed to experiment with exercise, explore my physical boundaries, and learn from my mistakes, all with minimal life obligations to deal with during the process.

It seemed simple, really. I'd start small and as my body gradually got stronger, I'd slowly ramp up my efforts from there. And when that exercise made me feel worse, I would take a break and rest and just wait until I felt better before continuing on with my exercise program. It wouldn't be *easy*, per se, but simple. As far as I was concerned, success with exercise was all about having absolute focus on my exercise plan and having the time to recover. When I'd tried and failed with exercise when I'd first gotten sick, I'd thought it was because I wasn't prepared to endure enough suffering. I'd given up too quickly. And during the years that followed, I chalked up my failures with exercise to having too many commitments. With responsibilities, I thought exercise was impossible. But with a clear calendar, I'd convinced myself that it was completely doable. I'd decided that once I carved out the time to focus on exercise, everything would be straightforward. This was my formula for escaping from the prison of CFS. And once I'd finally freed myself up from the demands of paying bills and keeping up with a full-time job, I thought I was home free. I was certain that after a few short months of dedication to my exercise-recover-repeat plan I would be marveling over my progress and euphoric over my newfound athletic abilities.

Yikes! Getting my body used to exercise again proved to be a much more difficult and complicated task than I ever could have anticipated. Maybe if I hadn't been sick and inactive for so long, this all might have gone a little bit better for me. Almost a decade of inactivity would take its toll on a healthy person, never mind a body battling CFS, so it seems safe to assume that I didn't do myself any favors by waiting that long to get active.

It turns out it wasn't just a matter of having the time to do it. Having a clear calendar certainly helped, but in the end that *wasn't* the lynchpin holding the whole exercise plan together. There were actually ways to significantly minimize downtime, but it took me a while to figure that out. And it wasn't just a matter of moving my body for a few minutes a day and watching my progress unfold. There was definitely more to that too.

Figuring out how much and what kind of exercise to do turned out to be more complicated than I'd expected. *Should I start with light cardio? Or strength training? How many days per week should I try to exercise?* It all felt quite confusing, and I soon realized that I had more questions than answers. I'd thought that I'd had a plan when it came to exercise, but really, I didn't.

It took me quite a while to learn how to make an exercise plan that worked well with CFS. I had to push myself enough to make progress, but I also needed to respect my body's limitations, not do damage, and, as much as possible, avoid setting myself back. It was an incredibly fine line to determine, and the penalties for misjudging that line could be huge.

Even though initially my workouts only lasted a couple minutes and I only did them every couple days, my body still seriously protested and caused me all kinds of grief. Beyond experiencing the typical muscle soreness that we all expect as a result of exercising, I had incredible aches all over my body. They came on mostly at night and felt like they went all the way down to my bones, making it incredibly difficult to sleep. And I desperately needed that sleep so that I could recover from these workouts, making the whole process even more frustrating and exhausting.

Regardless of how little exercise I did, I was always exhausted afterward, usually for the remainder of the day, and sometimes even for a couple days afterward. Once I'd started exercising I also got daily headaches that set in like clockwork right after dinnertime. I developed restless leg syndrome too — another serious yet absurd-sounding affliction to add to my list. If something has a title that makes it sound like a made-up bullshit condition, I've probably gotten it.

In short, I was doing very little exercise, yet suffering so much.

When I tell most people who don't have CFS that for me exercise was instrumental for recovery from CFS, I'm sure it sounds like a no-brainer. Most of us know that exercise is good for us. As I painstakingly learned, however, with CFS things get a bit complicated when it comes to exercise. If not done correctly, I've found that exercise can do incredible damage to the CFS sufferer, and I eventually learned that if I wanted to recover from my workouts and continue to get stronger, there were many things that I needed to do that a *regular* person didn't have to.

Eventually, I learned that there were ways I could support my body and speed up recovery. I didn't have to suffer so much, and I didn't have to give up quite so much either. I had to make exercise an absolute priority in my life, but I didn't have to be a slave to it. With the right approach and the right support for my body, it could all be manageable.

And I worked on changing my vocabulary. Since I found that the word *exercise* had become a dreaded four letter word of sorts, I started to think of it as *movement* instead. Movement felt intuitively healthy to me, and far less scary and intense than the dreaded 'e' word.

However, despite the vocabulary shift, in the beginning I definitely had a rough go of things. I was in a lot of pain and suffered quite a bit. I made progress, always at great personal cost. But with each passing month, as I experimented and found ways to make it all work better, things started to improve. The recovery process got more manageable. In time, I learned that it wasn't just about exercise, but about the diet, sleep, body support, schedule, and mindset that went with it.

Looking back I realize now that I didn't need to have waited for that perfect window of opportunity. If I knew then what I know now — what I'm sharing with you in this book — I could have fit movement into my routine. I'm not going to lie to you; if this is something that you and your doctor think you should take on, this will take a lot of effort and some serious focus. If it were easy, everyone would be doing it, and there'd be no need for this book. You will likely have to cut back on some things and make some modifications to your life, but waiting until circumstances are absolutely perfect isn't key. My earlier failed attempts convinced me I needed an all-or-nothing moment in my life to get better — so I put getting better on hold for years. I don't blame myself for waiting, but I wish I could get those years back. I'm sharing with you these insights so you don't have to wait for the "perfect" moment to get better. Start now, start small, and if your experience is anything like mine, eventually you'll get there.

If I could dial back the clock to Day One with CFS, this is what I'd tell myself about how to structure my life and support my body in the way that best supports an exercise (or movement!) program.

Building your body back up again will be serious business. You will make mistakes, push too hard, and crash and burn more times than you can count. As you learn how to slowly expand your body's limits, having a life that **permits you to crash** and fall on your face once in a while is essential. You'll need time to experiment and test your body's limits and figure out what works.

If you wake up the morning after exercise (that's when it always hit me the hardest) and can't get out of bed, that needs to be ok. You need to know that you can rest (guilt-free) as much as needed and that you aren't neglecting anything important in the process.

I know this sounds hard to accomplish. If you've got an

overflowing plate of responsibilities right now, you'll likely have to make some adjustments. If you're working, allot your vacation days for recovery time, and be at peace with using up that sick leave. If a full-time work schedule doesn't seem feasible even with those occasional days off, see if your doctor will support a temporary reduction in hours, or fill out the necessary paperwork for a short-term disability leave. Check if your employer offers disability insurance, because you might actually be able to retain all or some of your pay while on disability leave. If you are the full-time caregiver to your children, find some family members, friends, or paid helpers that can be on hand to step in and help out on the days that you need it. Take a look at your list of daily responsibilities and see where spouses, friends, family, and, if possible, some paid help can step in and take over some of the duties hanging over you.

And cut down on those demands that *you* place on *yourself.* Your hair, face, hands, and toes don't always have to be polished and perfect. Clothes don't always have to be ironed. The house doesn't always have to be spotless, and your meals don't need to be complex. The emails can wait, and you can skip the Christmas cards this year. Figure out what is *absolutely essential*, and then do only that.

I in no way mean to trivialize your obligations. I'm sure you have many important things that you need to do in your life, and cutting out or cutting back on any of them might just feel impossible. But to say that small changes will cure this illness is to trivialize CFS. What you choose to put in, and what you are able to put in, will likely directly translate into the degree of results that you see. It's an unfortunate and unfair reality. But lying and saying that putting in a small effort and not making your recovery your absolute priority will get you well isn't helping anyone either. I suspect that once again the misunderstood nature of this illness (combined with its crappy name) is working against us here. If you had cancer, neither you nor anyone else in your life would think twice about the appropriateness of your taking drastic measures and going all in on your healing plan. So take this seriously, and be that awesomely creative person that I know you are and think outside the box and find a way to simplify your life, make yourself a priority, and make this work for you.

Next, you need to focus on **what you *can* do** instead of focusing on what you can't. As a result, you'll be so much more excited when it comes time to exercise. No matter how small, it's *all* exercise. It's *all* progress. It *all* counts. As long as you're not pushing too hard or causing damage to your body, as long as you have the time carved out in your life to give yourself time to recover, know that your struggles aren't in vain and that it is all worth the effort you are putting in. Watch those small gains add up over time, and rejoice over the extra minute you add onto your workout each week. If you keep your eyes fixed on *these* things then you will see that the trajectory you are on is taking you someplace amazing.

For me, I'll be honest, this was incredibly hard to do. Before CFS I would look at a workout like a boot camp class, that would have been soul-sucking for most people, as just another day at the gym. And now I was telling myself that merely doing a few bicep curls with plastic-coated bubblegum-colored tiny little weights that look like they were designed for children was progress? But it was. Once I got myself in the mindset to stop seeing these minuscule weights in terms of my past but instead, in light of my future, those weights started to look pretty damn impressive. And those tiny weights led to the slightly bigger-sized dumbbells that were stored on the "real" workout rack, and then to the more impressive-sized ones farther down the stand, and over time — while I've yet to get back to boot camp — I began doing workouts that felt like genuine exercise.

Learning how to help your body recover turns out to be hugely important. Initially, your body might feel like it is raging against all forms of exercise. Physical activity, something that is supposed to be healthy and energizing for our bodies, can actually feel toxic to someone with CFS.

The days following my workouts could be absolute hell. Even the usual muscle pain that most people experience for a day or two after exercise could last up to five days for me, never mind all the other horrors I went through after just one quick trip to the gym. But over time I learned how to better support my body after exercise and speed up my recovery time. When my muscles were stretched, heated, and fully rested, they were happier and recovered much more quickly.

It's always good to **stretch** after workouts, but I've found that with CFS you have to take this activity to a whole other level. Since I'd always been in the habit of stretching after workouts in the past, I of course kept this practice up when I started my CFS recovery workouts. And in time I started to notice that with CFS, the more I stretched, the better I felt. With this illness, something happened in my body that made my muscles feel incredibly tight and tense most of the time, and all that stretching that suddenly came along with my workouts went a long way toward helping my body recover.

If you don't have the energy to both do some exercises and then stretch afterward, then in the beginning, if you can mage it — *just stretch*. If it's all you can manage, just stretch for a few minutes per day. Once your body gets used to that, then add some small strength-training exercises in the middle of your stretches. But no matter what, even if it's the only thing you do, the stretching has to happen.

In addition to stretching after my workouts, I also found it helpful to stretch every single night before I went to bed. If I didn't, it was pretty much guaranteed that I would have a long, sleepless night tossing and turning, trying to find a comfortable position in which my pain-filled body could rest. And if I woke in the middle of the night, I'd stretch some more. You don't even have to get out of bed if you find this happening to you. Simply sit up and do some simple stretches while still in bed, and you'll likely find that when you lie back down you'll quickly fall back asleep.

Even now that I'm recovered, I still stretch every night before I go to sleep. I have an alarm set on my phone that reminds me that it's time to get on my yoga mat for ten minutes and stretch out my body. As a result, my flexibility has improved, and my sleep is always better. Whether healthy or sick, as you stretch and relax your body you also relax your mind, which puts your whole self in a great space to get a good night's sleep.

Another savior for the CFS exerciser (if you can manage it) is hot water. In the beginning, while exercising with CFS I took so many **hot baths** that I thought I might never want to take another bath again ever in my life. But for a long time I couldn't live without them. Before soaking in the steamy tub, my whole body would be achy, restless, and just generally uncomfortable, but as soon as I got out, I would feel mostly pain-free and completely relaxed.

If you think your body can handle this, at a minimum, get

into hot water each night right before you go to bed. If you don't have a tub, then take a hot shower. Make this an ingrained part of your routine, something you know is essential in helping your muscles relax and recover and to getting the sleep you need.

And the hotter the water, the better the results. To be able to tolerate as hot of water as possible, get into the bathtub when it is still empty and then let the tub fill up while you are sitting in it. This way you can adjust to the heat as the tub fills, slowly increasing the temperature along the way (like a frog in a pot of boiling water — just be sure to get out before it's actually boiling!). And just like with the stretching, sometimes you might have to get up in the middle of the night to take yet another hot bath so that you can get back to sleep. You might not love all of this nocturnal stretching and bathing, but if you want your body to recover quicker, for a while this is what might need to happen.

Sleep at any cost. This needs to be your mantra.

I'm going to talk about this more in chapter 13, but it bears repeating. While recovering from CFS, you can't afford to lose any sleep unnecessarily. Whether this is due to someone else's snoring and movement in the night, or a brightly lit bedroom, steps need to be taken to ensure that you are getting the rest and recovery time you need. If your partner is keeping you up then one of you has to sleep somewhere else for a while. You might not love this, and you might not think that sleeping in separate rooms is the best thing for your relationship, but remind yourself of the long-term goal, which is to *make you better* — and that in the long run, making you better will make your relationship better too.

Take a look at the quality of sleep that you're getting, and if it's not optimal then change whatever needs to be changed. Get some earplugs and an eye mask or install some blackout blinds. Put a lock on your door so that people aren't coming in before you're ready to get up. Remove electronics from your sleep space, and invest in some new bedding that makes your bed feel like a welcoming and relaxing place to be. If your doctor feels it's appropriate, take some sedatives for a short while. Whatever you do, just make sure that you're getting in the hours that your body so desperately needs to recover.

I want to end this chapter by identifying two key counterintuitive outlooks that are going to be central to your success with exercise.

The first is that you need to **surrender to your limitations**. Continually pushing way past what your body is capable of will likely keep you sick forever. Understanding and appreciating this is absolutely essential. Take it from me: denial is not your friend here. Neither is the philosophy of *mind over matter*. CFS is not in your head! The physical limitations you are experiencing are very real. If two minutes of exercise is laying you out for days, then immediately dial it back to one minute. It's ok to test your limits and try different things to see what you are capable of, but you need to learn from your mistakes quickly. You need to fail fast and rapidly readjust your exercise program when you see that it is causing you more harm than good.

Learn to value consistency over intensity. If you need to start with only one minute of light exercise each day, then start there. Accept that this is where you are at and celebrate your commitment to doing it regularly. When this starts to feel a bit too easy, bump it up to two minutes per day. A little bit every day (or even every second day) will prove to be far more effective for you than one big workout that requires a few days or more of recovery time. Those down days when you can't exercise at all will really delay your overall progress, so not accepting your limitations will only ever serve to keep you from getting well. Once you finally commit to going small and to putting your ego aside, that's when you'll start making leaps and bounds toward your health goals.

The second attitude adjustment is to embrace the fact that **vanity cannot be your motivation**. Your goal cannot be to lose twenty pounds or attain six-pack abs or to impress people at the gym with your grueling workouts. Ignore that sad little number on the treadmill's display showing you the measly number of calories that you've burned after you've finished your workout. Burning calories is *not* your goal. Rest assured that you're gaining so much more from that time you just spent on the treadmill than the built-in display on the machine can ever show you. You'll be building up and strengthening every part of your body and doing so much amazing work that the limited software on the gym equipment unfortunately cannot measure or report.

Society has trained us to use calorie counts and our bathroom scale as our main indicators of success, but you need to leave these *numbers* behind for good. The progress you are making cannot be measured with a number. In their book *Younger Next Year*, authors Chris Crowley and Henry S. Lodge, MD, insist that the point of exercise is not to burn off calories, but rather to tell every part of your body to grow, to invest in building new tissue, and to run at a higher metabolic rate all day and all night long. Your one-minute workout, despite not changing any digital numbers, is all about doing "Number One" — you — a *tremendous* amount of good. And your goal, at least for now, is only healing from CFS, and that requires a different perspective from which to approach your exercise routine. Rest assured, even with putting vanity aside, the sexiest body you've ever had in your life is going to be waiting for you at the finish line, because when you're recovered from CFS, you'll feel in tune with your body instead of out of step with it, and that can't help but be expressed in the way you look. You'll be free from CFS and free from the tyranny of the mirror as well.

Now that we've covered the mindset required for a successful CFS recovery exercise plan, and you know how to best support your body during this process, in the next chapter, it's time to get into how to actually *do* the exercise. Because as they say, a goal without an actual plan is just a wish!

12

CARRYING OUT YOUR EXERCISE PROGRAM

When it comes to exercise programs and CFS, traditional mindsets like *more is better* and *always stay consistent* will not serve you well here. Just like with everything else involved with CFS recovery, when it comes to the actual *doing* of the exercise, there are some things that you need to pay close attention to and tailor to your specific needs. The typical "rules" for strength-training and cardio need to be modified, and there are some great resources available to help you quickly and easily design appropriate workouts for your recovery.

And this feels like a good time to remind you that what I'm sharing here is what worked *for me*. This is not a one size fits all exercise plan for CFS recovery and I absolutely am not saying that it will work for everyone. I know that when it comes to CFS, the topic of exercise is definitely a sensitive one. And with good reason because in my experience, too much exertion can do incredible damage to the CFS sufferer. But despite whatever past failed past attempts at working out you've had, I encourage you not to write off exercise immediately. Try to be open-minded with this topic while taking a serious look at the approach I've come up with. And then talk to your doctor and make an assessment regarding whether this might be right for you.

When it comes to exercise, I want to start by telling you what to avoid, and first and foremost on that list are **group fitness classes and personal trainers**. I can almost guarantee (at least initially) that group fitness classes and personal trainers can't provide you with what you need. It seems most doctors aren't even educated properly about CFS, so it's unlikely that personal trainers or fitness instructors will be either. Unless you are at a fitness center designed specifically for treating CFS patients, these fitness trainers likely can't understand the big picture or give you what you need to recover from this disease.

The pressure of trying to keep up with a group fitness class or the demands of an in-person trainer will cloud your ability to listen to your body and almost certainly keep you from scaling back as needed. Not even another person with CFS will know what is the right amount of exercise for you — only you will. (You'll notice that I'm **not** even going to provide you with a sample workout the way I did with food. Even I don't know what's going to be right for you!)

With well-intentioned fitness trainers in your face pushing you to work harder, it will be challenging to hear your body gently whispering to you and telling you when it is time to stop. And even if the fitness trainers aren't pushing you at all, something inside of you will likely still want to show that person — or group — how hard you are trying, which might cause you to push to do more than you are ready for.

It's only natural to want to finish an entire fitness class and keep up with the people around you. It's all too easy to lie to yourself and tell yourself that keeping up will be ok for you. In as little as one minute you can do too much. Just one minute! A miscalculation on your part that includes any exercise beyond what you are capable of could keep you in bed for the rest of the week. The price is too high and the voices from your body too easily ignored, so in the beginning, it's best to exercise on your own.

If you're not confident in your knowledge and ability to work out safely and effectively by yourself, book a *single session* with a personal trainer and have them design a workout for you to do alone. During this session you can share in detail the gentle nature of what you're looking for and they can teach you how to do the exercises safely and send you off to carry things out on your own time and at your own pace.

Think of your physical body as a body of water. And seeing as how humans are made up of mostly water, this analogy isn't much of a stretch. Bodies of water, when they keep moving, have a much better chance of staying healthy. But stagnant bodies of water are almost always breeding grounds for nastiness and disease. This is where any exercise program should start — simply with movement.

Our bodies have evolved to thrive in environments where we need to move and forage all the time, and that frequent movement is essential for our health and survival. In *Undo It!* Dr. Dean Ornish and Anne Ornish reveal that women who sit more than six hours per day are 37 percent more likely to die prematurely than those who sit fewer than three hours per day, even if they exercise regularly.

When we don't move our bodies regularly, we increase the risk of getting so many different illnesses. Part of the reason for this, according to these authors, is that our lymphatic system (our garbage removal system) can't do its work when we're not moving. On top of the lymphatic vessels, this system also includes important parts of our immune system such as our tonsils, appendix, thymus, and spleen. Whenever we are sedentary, this system can't transport vital infection-fighting white blood cells throughout our body.

Every time we move our bodies we send important "grow" signals to our body and mind, and when it comes to recovering from CFS, sending those signals just once a day isn't going to be enough. I know that with CFS the last thing you might feel up to doing is moving around often. And doing too much physical activity can definitely be damaging. The key here is to find ways to move your body as much and as often as you can without doing harm.

When CFS is quite bad, this might simply mean doing some simple arm and leg movements while in bed, or slowly swinging your arms around in circles every time you get up to go to the bathroom. And if you're up for it, on the way back pause in the hallway and do a couple squats. While you're on the couch or in bed, periodically lift your legs up and down and bend your limbs a bit. Set a timer on your phone to remind you to do this every thirty–sixty minutes, or however much you can manage. Whatever you do, it all counts, and it's all helping your body do what it needs to heal.

When you're ready to turn movement into directed exercise, it's time to find a workout that works for you. But if you shouldn't do classes or work with trainers, where can you turn? The **Internet** turns out to be an invaluable resource when it comes to exercise. Check out YouTube videos, download reputable fitness apps onto your phone, and get ideas for workouts from trustworthy websites and blogs. Some really great personal trainers have put their workouts into fitness apps, allowing you to still benefit from their knowledge and expertise *without* having the pressure to keep up with the programs they've designed exactly as they've designed them. The insights they have are terrific — it's their motivational techniques that people with CFS have to stay away from.

In the beginning your workouts will be really basic, consisting of simple exercises like a handful of squats or a few push-ups off of your knees. At this point, pretty much anything you do will likely help, because your whole body will desperately need work.

Once your workouts start getting longer, it can be a bit time consuming to have to keep designing your own effective workouts. To remedy this I use a great mobile app called Sweat that I absolutely love and still use to this day. It's not free, but I think it's a steal for receiving so many expertly designed workouts. It has a variety of workout options specifically designed for women (although I'm sure they'd work for all genders), and although I haven't tried it myself, there's a unisex app called Centr that I'm told is also great. What I love about apps like these (and about the Internet in general with respect to exercise) is the freedom you have to try different programs and find the best fit for you — with low entry barriers. Joining a health club is expensive; finding just the right trainer is time consuming. With the Internet, you can rapidly cycle through options until you find the right one for you with minimal time and outlay. And although you might still push too hard sometimes, overall I suspect you'll find it so much easier to turn off an app than to walk out mid-exercise class or to have to tell a personal trainer that you're quitting.

Using an app like Sweat means you don't have to spend any time at all designing your workouts, which frees up your precious energy for other (frankly more important) things. Each week Sweat has a new seven-day plan for you, warm-up and stretching included, that you can just plug and play as needed. It even has workout programs that don't require much equipment, meaning they can conveniently be completed from home.

Each trainer on Sweat also has a strong social media presence, so it's easy to connect with and follow others on platforms such as Instagram who are doing the program. Even if your progress is slower than some others, it is still really *encouraging* to see so many amazing people whipping themselves back into shape and fighting hard to regain their health. Social media definitely can give you a way to feel connected to others during a time when you don't have the energy to accomplish this in person. And lurking online reduces the pressure to be at the front of the class and overdoing it.

Indeed, in the beginning, the workouts in apps like this will more than likely be too tough for you, so you will have to modify them to make them easier. And for quite some time, even with these modifications, you will still have to cut the workouts in half, or thirds, taking two or three days to complete each workout with rest days in between. Remember, while you have to allow yourself time to crash, you should not aim for that as a goal!

Doing a modified version of the workouts the trainer put in the app means that you are still getting a balanced full-body workout — just at a much lighter and slower pace. Lower the number of repetitions and number of sets you do, and pause the app to take as many breaks as you need (again, another benefit of using an app versus a trainer or taking a class). If the app tells you to jump for an exercise, step it out instead. If push-ups are supposed to be from toes, do them from your knees. If the exercise calls for weights, use the absolute lightest weights possible, or just the bar — or even no weights at all.

If you aren't confident in your ability to modify a regular workout, then workouts designed for pregnant women can be a great option. These workouts are typically low intensity and don't involve excessively heavy lifting. When I was at the gym doing my super-light workouts, I'd sometimes remind myself that in that moment I actually wasn't all that different from a pregnant woman. My CFS body was growing somebody new inside of it — me! And because of this, for the time being, I had certain limitations and special accommodations that needed to be in place. CFS means you are dealing with some serious stuff, so give yourself permission to go easy. On the surface, with CFS we look like we should be able to do as much as everyone else, but we definitely can't. It's important to remind yourself of that when you're just starting out.

And as time goes on, you'll need to make fewer and fewer modifications and take fewer and fewer breaks. After so many years of struggling with CFS, these improvements with your strength will feel almost miraculous.

When I first started exercising, I gravitated toward light cardio activities such as walking on a treadmill or cycling gently on a recumbent bike. Although these activities felt the most manageable, they never really seemed to get me anywhere.

The best results I saw in recovering from CFS were by far from **strength training**. Once I mostly ditched the cardio and focused on strength training, my progress was much, much quicker. My energy started to increase faster, and my overall endurance for life got better.

When it comes to strength training with CFS, in the beginning this likely won't involve any weights. Stick to exercises like simple abdominal crunches or stationary lunges and anything else that gently works on *gaining* strength without straining your body too much. As you get stronger you can start incorporating the absolute lightest weights that the gym has into your workouts (optimally the one-kilogram/two-pound ones if they've got them).

Even in your weakened condition these tiny weights might feel too light for you, and as you lift them you might wonder how you could possibly be making any progress at all. When I used these small weights I honestly felt silly — like I was most likely wasting my time. But when I tried to go heavier, my health always crashed afterward. After going back to the smaller weights and trusting what my *body* was telling me (and not my mind), I discovered — much to my surprise — that with these small weights I was making tons of progress! And eventually I was able to increase to heavier weights *and* still feel good after my workouts.

I also found that full-body exercises that focused on natural motions such as mountain climbers, commandos, inchworms, bear crawls, and burpees really helped propel me toward my goals. If you don't know what these things are, don't worry — the exercise apps out there will teach you exactly how to do them!

This type of whole-body exercise is known in the workout world as calisthenics — an activity that uses minimal to no weights so that you can master your own bodyweight. It represents exercise in its most natural form and combines strength training with basic gymnastic movements that can be done almost anywhere.[1] Cross training is another whole-body workout approach that includes aerobics, flexibility training, and weight training that could work well for CFS recovery.[2] In my experience, Yoga, with its focus on flexibility and gentle whole-body strengthening, has its place also. The spiritual and mental aspects of this form of exercise would most definitely benefit the CFS sufferer, but for purely physical training, supplementing your yoga practice with some additional strength training would likely speed up your overall CFS healing process.

Circuit training is another option for CFS recovery. When done as designed, it involves rapidly moving from one exercise to the next. Apps such as Sweat offer up circuit training options, and I think they can work great for CFS recovery if the breaks between exercises are significantly lengthened (meaning it's no longer really circuit training by definition) — but if you're not concerned about the label, the workouts will still work for you.

Plyometrics, with its nickname of *jump training,* should make it obvious that this one will have to wait until you are further down your CFS recovery journey, because early on the explosive high-intensity movements will almost certainly earn you a couple days in bed. And isometric exercises (whose name also gives them away), with their focus on small muscle groups, is not ideal for CFS recovery. It does not effectively build strength and is best suited for healing a specific part of your body (say, for instance, a rotator cuff) than it is for healing a full-body chronic illness such as CFS.[3] Pilates exercises focus primarily on the core muscles and not so much on the rest, so these types of targeted workouts should also be reserved for further down the line.

In time, all of these workouts can have something to offer your CFS recovery journey. As long as you initially stick to gentle full-body workouts that are done on your own, you can eventually switch it up to other exercise approaches and even join some group classes when you feel you are ready. It's all about knowing what works best when, and not shooting yourself in the foot by doing things that are working against your body instead of with it.

I think **cardio** definitely has its place in an exercise regimen, just not during the early recovery days with CFS. As your health improves and you feel like you have energy to spare after your strength-training workouts, you can try spending a few minutes walking on the treadmill. Walking is such a natural movement for humans, and I think that when possible getting in a few steps each day is important. Eventually you will benefit from bringing regular cardio sessions back into your life.

When it comes to cardio, just as with the strength training, if your experience is anything like mine then you're going to have to start really small. You might think that because you've built up some strength and are actually using some impressive-sized weights at the gym that you'll be able to jump in and do a quick fun run. But this is unfortunately **not** the case — be prepared for a major setback if you try that. Whether it's running or swimming or biking, whatever you chose will be a whole other ballgame for your body, and you'll have to work on getting it used to this new activity very slowly.

Start with just a few *minutes* of low-intensity cardio. When you feel ready, start adding a couple thirty-*second* segments of higher intensity. Each week, try adding a couple more thirty-second segments. Because you've already done quite a bit of conditioning with the strength training, you'll likely see much faster improvements with cardio than you initially did with the weights. It might feel a little like you're starting all over again, but be patient, and before you know it that fun run should be no problem at all.

Few things in life make me happier than having a plan and sticking to it, but in the beginning, no matter how hard I tried, I could almost never stick to my exercise plan. Week after week I'd make a rigid exercise schedule, and week after week I'd feel like a failure when I wouldn't be able to follow it.

With CFS, having a plan is important, but so is having some serious **flexibility** with that plan. (And if this Master Planner over here is saying that then you know it must be true!) That line between not doing enough exercise and doing too much is so fine that I don't think that even someone with rock-solid self-discipline could manage never to cross it. And the unfortunate reality is that, usually, the only way to discover what your limits are is to occasionally pass them. In the beginning, it's likely that you'll frequently need more days off for recovery than planned, and because of this, you're going to have to be prepared to be flexible and adapt your schedule as you go.

Just remember that no matter how small your workouts might feel, they are actually giant steps toward getting your health back and experiencing genuine freedom. It's all exercise, it all counts, and it's all infinitely better than doing nothing.

If you're one of those people who doesn't get very pumped up at the thought of exercise, don't worry; in time that will change. As explained by Crowley and Lodge, as you get into better shape and get stronger, your brain will secrete more adrenaline when you exercise. You will actually start to enjoy the weights and look forward to going to the gym.

So if the thought of embarking on this exercise program isn't exactly thrilling, hang in there, because whether you believe it now or not, soon you will be grinning ear to ear while you work out and gleefully posting sweaty gym selfies on social media like a fool.

13

BECOMING YOUR BODY'S ALLY

I like to think of myself as my body's personal assistant, dutifully bringing it the things it needs to function effectively and eliminating the things that keep it from getting its work done. When I take care of my body and support the ways in which it heals and maintains itself, it's amazing what it accomplishes. Our bodies are miraculous and, if treated properly, are often better than any doctor at healing themselves when they are injured. The best thing we can do for our bodies is to make sure they are getting what they need to get their work done.

Over the years I've tried countless cleanses and detoxes where I'd consume various shakes and herbal potions, pop handfuls of supplements, and basically do whatever the latest cleansing book or blog told me to do, and all I've taken away from these experiences is that for me, these types of cleanses don't work. I'm just not convinced there's anything that you can put into your body to clean it.

But I have found, as with the case of periodic fasting, that there are things that you can do to support your body's *own* ability to cleanse and heal itself. There are some things that, when done regularly, without fail help my body thrive. If I'm feeling off, sluggish, or ill in any way, I take a look and see what I've been neglecting, or in what area I might have to ramp up to help my body heal.

Is there anything that we do for our bodies that makes us feel better than **sleep**? Sometimes a good night's sleep feels like it can fix almost anything. And if I'm having an especially rough day, a nap can almost always completely turn that around.

Most of us love to sleep, and there's a reason for that. The way you feel while you're awake depends in part on what happens while you're sleeping. During sleep, your body is working to support healthy brain function and maintain your physical health.[1] In order for your body to be able to do the magnificent things it does to heal and rejuvenate itself, it absolutely needs adequate good-quality sleep. Sleep is involved in the healing and repairing of your heart and blood vessels and in decreasing the risk of obesity. While we sleep our bodies also release hormones that boost muscle mass and help repair cells and tissues.[2] People who get enough sleep also have more energy, get sick less often, lower their risks for heart disease and diabetes, experience reduced stress and improved mood, think more clearly, and just generally get along better with others.[3] Besides robbing you of energy and time for muscle repair, lack of sleep saps your motivation, which is a huge problem — because motivation is what's needed to keep going and get yourself to the finish line when you are recovering from CFS.

Without sufficient sleep, I'm positive I never would have recovered from CFS, because the healing and repair that takes place while I'm sleeping is significant and seems impossible to replicate with anything else.

To heal from CFS, I'm convinced you need to get some sleep at whatever cost necessary. No price is too high.

What does this mean? This means that if you're not getting enough sleep, you might have to consider doing some things that you wouldn't normally want to do so that you can increase the amount of sleep that you're getting.

I'm not a great sleeper under the best of circumstances, so getting enough shut-eye while struggling with CFS was especially challenging for me. And the worse my CFS symptoms were, the worse my sleep was. It's frustrating that the times when our bodies need sleep the most are the times we often struggle the most to get it.

I don't know about you, but I am happiest when I get up at the same time every morning (the earlier the better) and go to bed at the same time every night. As someone who typically struggles to get a good night's sleep, this consistency not only makes me happier but helps me sleep better too. Plus, there's just something about being up early each day that can make me feel on top of my life and generally just good about the day ahead.

But with CFS, you might have to abandon the practice of both being up early and being up at the same time every day. While sick, the amount of sleep needed from night to night can be inconsistent, which makes following any set schedule challenging. When your symptoms are especially bad, I've found you might need as much as fourteen hours of sleep in a single night. If you have a bad couple nights where you don't get much sleep at all, there is no moving forward with your life until that sleep debt is repaid. Some days, if your body demands it, you might not be up before noon. You might not love this, but I've found it's the only way to respond to your body's varying levels of fatigue and give it the rest it needs.

My body also struggled if I tried to make sudden or drastic

changes to my sleep pattern. If I woke up at noon one day, it would be incredibly hard on my body to try and get up at 9:00 a.m. the next. This meant that after sleeping late one day, it could take a while to get myself to a place where I could comfortably get up early again.

With CFS, being gentle is key. When possible, never get up more than one hour earlier than you did the day before. If you get up at noon one day, set your alarm for 11:00 a.m. the next day, and then 10:00 a.m. the day after that, and so on. Sudden changes seem to wreak havoc on bodies suffering from CFS and make you feel even more terrible than you usually do, so try to make the changes to your sleep schedule as gradual as possible.

As I touched on earlier, even if you don't love the idea of sleeping in a separate bedroom from your partner, for a while, this also might be what needs to happen. If your doctor is on board, you might also have to come to terms with taking some sedative medications if you're finding that, despite making all the other changes, you still aren't getting sufficient good-quality sleep. And if you can afford it, upgrading to a comfortable high-quality bed can be beneficial as well.

On top of the CFS-specific sleep protocols that you follow, be sure to abide by conventionally recommended practices for improving sleep as well. Avoid sugar and alcohol, because their consumption pretty much guarantees a terrible night's sleep. And don't eat large meals or drink too many fluids too close to bedtime to ensure your body is not taxed with dealing with these items while attempting to rest.

And even when you can't maintain a consistent bedtime, maintain a consistent bedtime routine. Keep your bedroom dark and cool and free from brightly lit digital screens. Use natural good-quality lavender oils on your pillows to help you relax, and use an eye mask and earplugs to cut down on extra light and noise. I know that some people don't find that reading in bed helps them, but I find that reading a light and relaxing book on my dimly lit Kindle is always an effective way to shut my mind down and allow sleepiness to take over. Short, nightly meditations also help clear your mind, let go of the day, and prepare to sleep.

With CFS, I've found that naps are also your best friend. If you feel the need to sleep during the day, don't hold back. When my health was at its worst I napped *every single day.* Sometimes twice. I usually didn't set any kind of an alarm, which meant I often played a kind of nap roulette in which I never knew how long I was going to sleep. I might wake up in twenty minutes or in four hours — it was anybody's guess. But it's important to let your body decide how much sleep it needs, so stay away from setting alarms as much as possible.

When it comes to CFS, anything and everything that might help you sleep better must be considered, because getting that high-quality restorative sleep each and every night is so important for getting better. This isn't the time to please others and worry about what they think. This isn't the time to judge yourself and expect yourself to do everything without any help. Try different things, do what's needed, and don't stop experimenting until you are sleeping at least eight solid hours each and every night. This is when your body is doing the most cleansing and repairing, and you need to make sure you are doing everything you can to ensure your body is getting as much of this essential healing time as it needs.

We seem to be a bit afraid of the **sun** these days, to the point where the word has almost become a bad word. The sun's gotten quite a bad rap, which is unfortunate because I know my body just sings when it gets even the smallest doses of it. Moderate sun exposure can bring important health benefits such as stronger bones, better sleep, improved mood, and a healthier immune system.[4] Research from Harvard Medical School shows that many people have low vitamin D levels from lack of sun exposure and that there is a well-documented relationship between low vitamin D levels and poor bone health, as well as links to multiple sclerosis and prostate cancer, among other conditions.[5] So when you continuously shield yourself from the sun or always cover every inch of exposed skin with sunscreen, you could be missing out.[6]

I'm not saying that we don't need to be careful when it comes to the sun. With the increasing intensity of our sun exposure, it seems we definitely need to limit our sunbathing. But the keyword here is *limit*, not *omit*. Yes, those days of gleefully baking in the sun for hours should probably be a thing of the past for all of us. There are real risks to our health from getting too much sun exposure, and it's great that there is so much awareness around this these days. But it seems we've gotten a bit too afraid of the sun and that removing it from our lives entirely is not the best for our health either.

So when possible, make spending some time in the sun a part of your daily routine. By doing so, you likely will find that your mood lifts and you feel better, look better, and sleep better. Even if it's a cloudy day, still go spend some time outdoors because some healing sunshine is still making its way through those clouds, and your body is still drinking up what it needs.

Despite all the crap we expose our bodies to — pollution, chemicals, junk food, drugs, alcohol, harmful bacteria, viruses, and a whole host of other stuff — it's amazing how it somehow manages to deal with most of it.

This is no small job for our bodies, and I've come to appreciate the huge role our **lymphatic system** plays in this cleaning job. The lymphatic system is a network of tissues and organs that helps rid the body of toxins, waste, and other unwanted materials. Its primary function is to transport lymph — a fluid containing infection-fighting white blood cells — throughout the body.[7] It essentially carries toxins and waste away from our tissues and into our bloodstream so that they can then be dealt with by the appropriate organs and eliminated.

The best thing for our bodies would obviously be to make sure that no toxins got in there in the first place, but unfortunately this is just not realistic. But what we *can* do is take measures to reduce our body's toxic load. As much as possible, we can keep processed foods, artificially scented candles, air fresheners, toxic hair and body products, cosmetics, perfumes, cleaning products, and so on out of our lives.

But as hard as we try, there's just no way to avoid all forms of toxicity. The good news is that, in my experience, you don't have to live inside an organic toxin-free bubble in order to recover from chronic fatigue syndrome. I did the bulk of my healing from CFS while living in a city in a developing country with some of the *worst* air pollution in the world — a place where on many days the smog was so thick you could see it. Your environment doesn't have to be perfect. Just eliminate what toxins you can while doing everything you can to support your body's detoxification abilities, and you will be amazed at what your body can accomplish.

Since the lymphatic system doesn't have its own pump (like our blood does), the biggest thing you can do is to help keep this fluid moving. One way we accomplish this is simply by moving. Every time we move our bodies, our lymph starts moving too. But when we don't have the energy to move all that much, another great way to get lymph flowing is by exposing ourselves to **alternating hot and cold water**. This causes the lymph vessels to dilate and contract, which also gets this vital fluid going.

Have you ever noticed that if you're feeling unwell, after jumping into a cold ocean or pool you often feel better afterward? It's amazing how much this simple activity can help. But what if you don't happen to conveniently have a chilly ocean or a swimming pool nearby to pop into each day?

Thankfully there are simpler and more convenient ways to get your body exposed to some cold water. The easiest way to accomplish this is to incorporate a new cold water habit into one of your existing routines: your shower. Every time you take a shower (if you think your body can manage this), simply turn the faucet to make the water as cold as you can manage it for one to two minutes. To make sure you remember, pair this activity with a specific part of your shower — say, when you rinse out your shampoo. While you are getting all those suds out simply turn the water from hot to cold and keep it there until you are finished with this stage of your shower routine. Thoroughly rinse your hair, face, and body to ensure all parts of you get exposed to the colder water temperature.

If you live in a hot climate, you can put the water setting to as cold as it will go and it will likely still be a comfortable temperature, but if you live in a colder climate you might have to play around a bit and see how cold you can comfortably manage. After your one- to two-minute cold blast, simply turn the water back up to a warmer temperature and finish the rest of your shower.

Some days, even though your one- to two-minute cold blast is finished, you might find that you want to keep it going longer. Some days your body might be thriving in the cooler water, and you actually will have no desire to turn the lever back to hot. So don't — in these instances you can almost hear your body speak out loud to you, insisting you give it more cold water. During these times it seems safe to assume that your body has a larger load of stuff to deal with, so it asks you (by sending you feelings of pleasure and happiness when you're in the cold water) to keep the cold shower going as long as possible.

In this toxin-laden world we live in, this cold water habit is good practice for both the sick and the healthy. And like anything, after you've done it for a while it will become so routine that you'll barely notice that you're doing it.

Another way to help your body's lymphatic system to maintain peak performance is to get regular full-body **massages**. I've found that deep-tissue full-body massages are invaluable in helping my body heal and feel its best. And the stronger the massage, the better I feel. At the start of any massage I always ask the therapist to go as hard as she can. It can be a bit of a painful experience sometimes, but as long as it's *good pain*, I don't mind it one bit. Of course this won't be suitable for everyone, and only you will know if you can handle massages and what intensity they should be. But for those who can manage it, I've found massages to be a great addition to an overall body healing support program.

Some places offer something called a *lymphatic drainage massage*, and although the title makes you think it should be the best for helping your lymphatic system, I often don't feel that much better after these massages. If you can manage it, the ones with names like *sports massage* or *deep-tissue massage* are usually the ones from which I get the most benefit. Perhaps it's because these deep-tissue massages are benefitting us in ways beyond supporting our lymphatic system. Whatever the reason, the strong massages always fix me right up.

I'm lucky in that some places that I've lived the massages have been quite cheap, so I was able to go for them often. Other places I've lived the massages were a bit more costly, so unfortunately I couldn't go as often. But I still go as much as I can.

Don't think of massages as a luxury or as some sort of self-pampering activity, but instead as a medically necessary part of your healing regimen. Budget for them, and do not feel guilty about the money you spend. It's an investment in yourself. Group the cost of massages into the same category in your budget as you do doctor's appointments and other medical costs. They are a vital component of your healing plan — don't skimp on them.

If your budget won't allow you to get quite as many massages as you would like, you can supplement your massage treatments with at-home stretching and foam roller exercises that will also get your lymphatic fluid flowing. There are many great mobile apps such as Sweat and many other websites that can guide you through some routines to help you stretch out your body and get things moving. Some massage therapists can even suggest stretches to do between sessions to tide you over. Just do what you can, as often as you can, and your body and future self will thank you.

Your body is giving you important messages at every moment of every day and, the more you listen, the better you'll be at being your body's personal assistant. Pain is information, and it's amazing what we can accomplish when we listen and respond to what our body is telling us. Is your body singing when exposed to cool water or the sun? Then it probably wants a bit more of it. Do you feel energized after a workout? Then you are most likely on the right track. But if your workouts leave you feeling overly exhausted and depleted, then your body is telling you to dial it back. The suffering we experience need not be in vain. The pain and discomfort are there for a reason, and we need to figure out what that reason is.

With CFS, your body is often overloaded and lacking the energy to heal itself. So on the days that it's especially hard to get out of bed, that's its way of telling you to give it a break. To possibly skip some meals and get some rest. To stop flooding it with toxic chemicals and harmful food and poisoning it with drugs and alcohol. It's asking you to let it rest and heal, so stop pushing beyond your limits and support your body in this process. Get on the same team as your body and help it escape CFS, because paying attention to what it needs is your way out of this prison.

VI

EMOTIONAL
EMANCIPATION

14

OVERCOMING A NEGATIVE MINDSET

Staying positive while suffering from CFS can feel a bit like trying to keep a smile on your face while getting poked with a searing-hot stick all day long. There isn't a moment where you don't have something challenging to deal with, and keeping your spirits up can sometimes feel impossible.

There were some days with CFS when everything just felt too difficult, days where I was flooded with feelings of sadness and fear and anger and depression and grief. Days where I was crying (again) for the zillionth time. Days where I felt that the suffering would never end and that not a single soul on the planet understood what I was going through.

When times were especially tough I had to use the bulk of my energy just to try and stay two steps ahead of a deep depression, one that threatened to keep me in bed for days on end if I let it catch me. I wish I could say that at every moment with CFS I was this unstoppable force that kept my eye on the prize no matter what, but unfortunately that wasn't always the case. Sometimes I felt truly beat down and completely defeated.

For instance, when I was living in Malaysia and already a

few years into my journey with CFS, I decided to go on a short holiday to a nearby island with some friends. Looking back, I have absolutely no idea why I agreed to go because this was not too long after I'd quit my exhausting teaching job and my body was in a really bad place. At that point in my journey, I'd often been in denial about my physical limitations and thought that mind over matter could get me through. Sometimes it could, but mostly it couldn't. For this trip, it turned out it definitely could not.

I woke up that first morning of that vacation on this stunning, textbook-tropical island, and I was so sick and bone-tired that I could barely get out of bed. I didn't even join the group for breakfast and ended up having to spend the whole day in bed in my hotel room while everyone else hung out at the beach, having fun and soaking up the glorious tropical sunshine.

At this point, I'd already been struggling with my health for years, and my first attempt back at working full-time had set my health back big time. My depression was intense and my tolerance for suffering depleted. I was so exhausted from the struggle of it all and I felt like I had truly run out of fight. I really didn't feel like I could keep doing it anymore. I was tired of everything always being so hard. I was tired of having to continually keep pulling myself back up again. I was tired of not being able to live life in the same capacity that most of the people around me could. Basically, I was tired of being sick and tired.

As I lay in bed that day in that hotel room, I started to fantasize — not about being able to go out and join my friends, but instead about lying alone on some deserted corner of the island and taking my own life. I desperately wanted to live, but I also wanted the suffering to stop. I *needed* it to stop. As I laid there imagining my life slipping away and leaving my body, the thought brought me so much peace. After years of CFS repeatedly defeating me, I felt hopeless and helpless and just wanted it all to finally be over. I could feel how my mother's heart would break if she knew that I, too, got to that level of immense suffering and total despair — that feeling that she knew all too well. But I felt like I had nothing left — no fight left in me. The finish line that I'd been chasing was starting to feel imaginary, and I didn't know how much longer I could keep chasing a fictitious dream. At the time the thought of all my struggles finally coming to an end in such a beautiful and serene spot really felt like it might be the best thing for me.

I struggled when trying to decide whether or not to include stories such as this one, because it's important to me that this be an uplifting and inspiring book about overcoming CFS. It's also not a great feeling putting such a raw and vulnerable piece of myself out into the world for public consumption.

But I also think that it's important to tell the *real* story of CFS, the whole story of what it was like for me because this can be a devastating, life-shattering disease that needs to be taken incredibly seriously at every stage of the illness. Ultimately, I decided that glossing over the ugly parts would be a disservice to CFS sufferers. By skipping over some of the harsher realities of this illness, people who don't have CFS can never hope to understand how devastating of an illness this really can be, and it also wouldn't show the people who have it that these feelings can be normal and that it's understandable if they too sometimes feel this low.

If you find yourself ever feeling like things have gotten so bad that you are contemplating taking your own life, you *have* to reach out to someone for help. Immediately call a friend or family member or go see a counselor. In Canada, you can text CONNECT (for English) or PARLER (for French) to 686868 to reach the Crisis Text Line. You can also dial 911 to be connected with the suicide and crisis hotlines in your specific province or territory. In the US you can call the National Suicide Prevention Hotline at 1-800-273-8255, or text CONNECT to 741741. Wikipedia also has a comprehensive list of global crisis lines that can be found at https://en.wikipedia.org/wiki/List_of_suicide_crisis_lines.

Thankfully, despite the deep depression I experienced while on that tropical island, I managed to find a way to keep pushing forward. I should have talked to someone, but I was too ashamed of how I was feeling to reach out. Mostly what got me through was thinking of what my death would do to my father. The only thought worse than continuing on with my suffering was the idea of putting him through the pain of the loss of his only child, and the repetition of a terribly traumatic pattern. So as I lay in bed, I read my books, and I distracted myself long enough for the deep depression to pass. And as always, once I physically started feeling the tiniest bit better, emotionally I started to perk up a bit as well, and things started feeling somewhat manageable once again.

The most important thing I got out of these moments was that they helped me appreciate that ignoring my emotional health just wasn't an option, and they pushed me to find strategies for how to better cope with CFS.

After hearing that story it'll come as no shock to hear that the first thing I would encourage you to avoid is negative thoughts. I know that sounds easier said than done, but start small. For example, as much as I love to educate myself about this illness, I've found that reading too much on the topic of chronic fatigue syndrome often left me feeling quite hopeless. Despite there being some documented cases of people who have completely recovered from CFS, most of the articles and books out there seem to focus mainly on how almost no one ever gets better from this mysterious disease. Most of what's out there in the news and media focuses on how the medical world just isn't equipped to deal with chronic illness in general, and taking in too much of that kind of information is emotionally counterproductive.

I have to be honest as well and say that I wouldn't have written this book if I'd already found a good one out there on CFS. I certainly haven't read everything, and some of what I have read did offer some small amounts of insight, but from my research much of the literature on CFS in book format seems quite repetitive. It seems as if many authors have read the same couple books and then just wrote more books repeating that same content. It can be frustrating and a waste of time to spend hours reading the same information over and over again, so after you feel that you've gotten the gist of most of what is out there, I'd put those books down.

My suggestion when it comes to CFS and health research in general is to, every once in a while, take a peek and see if there is anything that appears to be new or groundbreaking out there, and if there's not, shut down your search and switch to more helpful and inspirational sources of reading. Put some trust in everything you've already learned and use that to drive your healing efforts.

———

At the opposite end of the spectrum from hopelessness is having expectations that are just unrealistically optimistic. Much of the time our life isn't the problem; our expectations are. If we expect every single day of our lives to be perfect, then every time a bad day comes along we will be infuriated at the injustice of it, and we'll generally just be in for a rough ride in life. Whether you have CFS or not, the bad days are coming, and expecting and accepting them can make them so much easier to deal with.

It's like being in a relationship and expecting your partner to always be perfect, and then being shocked and frustrated every single time they aren't. If we modify our relationship expectations to a more reasonable level, then when these inevitable moments of imperfection come we can remind ourselves that sometimes our partners will be selfish, and sometimes they will say inconsiderate things, and this is just one of those times. They, like us, are human, and we can't expect them to be perfect for every single second of their lives.

When we expect these moments of imperfection, whether it be in relationships or in healing from CFS, it doesn't mean that these times don't sometimes still stir up some unpleasant emotions in us. It just means that we can more quickly put these events into perspective, with the intensity of these emotions diminished to a level that we can more easily deal with.

With CFS, when the bad days come, remind yourself that you knew that these days were coming and that they are an inevitable part of the healing process. On these bad days, use distraction. To take your mind off things, enjoy a favorite (healthy) food, ask a friend to come over for tea, get lost in some guided meditations, or binge-watch a favorite TV series. Do whatever you can to keep your mind busy and happy until the bad day has passed and you can start fresh again the next day.

And while struggling with CFS, managing the good days appropriately is just as important as managing the bad ones.

Throughout my CFS journey there were sometimes beautiful, blissful days where I felt almost like the *old me* — energetic and ready and able to take on the world. And sometimes, on these days, I did. I'd run errands and organize my closets and do enough food prep to last me a month. From dawn until dusk I would buzz around like a happy, energetic little bee doing all the things I'd longed to do on my sicker days but couldn't.

Holding back when you feel well, especially when it happens so infrequently, can be a huge ask. But I've paid some heavy prices over the years for my good days, so I quickly learned that on these days I really needed to take it easy. If you don't, it's sort of like burning through an entire paycheck on the first day you get it. It's fun for that day, but you will struggle every day after until you get paid again. So take it easy, and don't let one good day turn into a world of pain afterward.

In her *Psychology Today* article "Saving Your Own Life," Clinical Psychologist Georgia Witkin emphasizes that if you falter in life, remember that expecting too much of yourself can be unrealistic and even cruel. So ease up on yourself because you are doing great. In your most challenging times, talk to yourself the way you would talk to a friend. Imagine what you would say to someone you love who was facing what you're facing. Would you be critical? Or tell them to give up? Doubtful. I'm guessing you would give them a hug, remind them how wonderfully brave they are, and tell them how much they inspire you.

Do this for yourself as well, because you deserve it.

––––––––

This point goes hand-in-hand with my next one. If you're riding a horse and it dies, you need to get off.

In those early days with CFS, as I drained my bank

accounts and devoted the bulk of my days to my healing plan, I'd tell anyone who asked that my healing regimen was definitely working. Even when it wasn't. To keep from completely falling apart, regardless of how bad I was feeling, I'd usually plaster a smile on my face and pretend that, for the most part, everything was ok.

I wasn't lying, exactly. Not to them anyway; only to myself. I'd stubbornly and blindly keep riding that dead horse for months before I'd admit to myself what was going on, before I'd admit that what I was doing wasn't working and that I needed a new plan. My being an eternal optimist was blinding me to the facts and actually hindering my progress.

This was a definite low point for me, but it was a much-needed turning point as well. I learned that even though I might not always like what I saw, I needed to take off the blinders and make sure I was objectively assessing my progress. If my efforts were failing, I needed to learn to fail fast. I had to find the faults in my healing plan quickly and adjust accordingly.

The first time I admitted to myself that my whole plan to get well wasn't working, I actually crawled into my bedroom closet and started to cry. I just wanted the whole world to disappear while I crumbled in defeat. After all the money I'd spent and all the effort I'd put in, the realization that I wasn't getting better was devastating.

As important as it is to keep your sights on the good stuff in life, you also need to acknowledge and process the bad as well, because pretending that everything is fine all the time when it isn't doesn't serve anyone. It can be a bit challenging to determine where that healthy line is between staying positive and admitting things are crappy, and in all those awesome efforts to stay positive you've likely pushed a few negative emotions down along that way that should have been let out.

The easiest and most effective way I've found to deal with this backlog of negative emotions is to, every now and then, have a good cry. It's unbelievable what an effective release this can be! If I've let too much build up inside, once I start crying I usually find that there were quite a few tears waiting to be let out. I'm sure we've all experienced this before. You're watching a movie or a TV show and a sad part comes on and what starts as a normal and expected amount of tears for a fictional TV story quickly spirals into something completely disproportional to the situation at hand. Fifteen minutes pass and you're still doing the ugly cry. The bad news is that your face is now a red and swollen hot mess, but the good news is that your backlog of emotions needing a release has largely been taken care of.

Sometimes, when needed, these tears will come out all on their own. Other times, you know they're there, but for whatever reason, they need a little coaxing. If they need a little help to come out, pop on *The Notebook* or *Titanic* or *The Fault in Our Stars* or whatever tearjerker always makes you cry. Take that time to get lost in the sadness and let your waterworks fly because it truly is cathartic.

When negative emotions come up, notice them, feel them, fully experience them, and then let them pass. Like the rest of us, they just want a little bit of acknowledgment and appreciation for their existence. Once they get it, they'll chill out and leave you in peace.

Once you've had that cry you'll be asking yourself, "How do I look at myself without blinders? To think about CFS without getting too low as a result?" I recommend starting by imagining yourself as an anthropologist tasked with studying your own behavior. As a scientist, you'll be an objective, non-judgmental observer on a fact-gathering mission. Your only goal is to notice your habits and observe them, without judging them as good or bad. Regard yourself simply with curiosity. There is no right or wrong in what you see, only neutral observations of your behavior.

What I notice most about myself is that when I'm not acting the way I would like, perhaps by not reaching my expectations or sticking to my healthy diet, I get all judgmental and hard on myself. I get stuck in a state of self-blame and shame and from this place it can be really hard to figure out how to get onto a better path. Yet I've come to realize that being hard on myself does not serve me in any way. It's taken me quite a while to get to this place. I found it surprisingly difficult to let go of the self-hatred and self-punishment I seemed to love doling out on myself every time I "screwed up." But without fail, serving myself up all that negativity never helped one bit and almost always led to even more "bad" behavior.

When you beat yourself up and when you're feeling like crap about yourself you don't usually feel inspired to go out and make better decisions. You feel like sulking. Perhaps you eat an entire pizza or polish off a bottle of wine to try to make yourself feel better. Perhaps you do both. Maybe to lift your spirits you spend money you can't actually spare on some new clothes. Whatever it is, it usually just sets you back even further.

When your life isn't going the way you'd like, instead of beating yourself up over it, try being curious about what's going on. Treat your problem like a puzzle that you need to solve. So you planned to go to the gym three times this week and you didn't end up going even once. Chances are, the reason you didn't go is not because you're a lazy, unreliable, or bad person, and telling yourself this will not help you one bit. It's more likely that you didn't make it to the gym because something in your life is not structured in a way that supports your gym routine. Maybe you lacked a specific plan for when you would go. Perhaps you need to schedule the workouts in your calendar, and then leave your gym bag by the front door as an additional reminder. Maybe three times a week actually isn't realistic for you right now, and by setting too lofty of a goal you only made the plan overwhelming and unknowingly set yourself up to fail. Instead of being hard on yourself, examine your actions from a place of curiosity, and make your new plan of action from what you see.

This is the first step to emotional well-being: freeing your mind from negative thoughts. Doing so isn't easy, but in the end, it will make you feel so much lighter and you will have taken a giant leap toward being the resilient, resourceful, and happy person that we all are striving to be. It's sort of like restarting your computer — by ridding yourself of your toxic thought patterns you're hitting the reset button, cleaning out the bugs that have been accumulating in the shadows, and getting yourself ready to tackle what you're about to accomplish next. Once free from negativity, your mind is no longer bogged down and it has the space it needs to develop the new habits and ways of thinking that will lead you toward health and happiness.

15

BALANCING YOUR EMOTIONS

We often hear that happiness in life comes in waves, but the part that is left out in this metaphor is that if happiness is the wave, then we are the surfer. It's up to us to stand and catch those waves; otherwise, all that happiness will just keep passing us by. There's some effort involved, but the payout is more than worth it.

If you want to be happy, you have to be happy *on purpose*. Life coach Jordana Jaffe urges that every day of your life can be the best or the worst day of your life — it's all about the evidence you're looking for to support either one. The more you look for things to be grateful for, the happier you'll be.

Sometimes with CFS it can feel like the struggles will never end, and it can be tempting to lose faith and want to throw in the towel. But chances are that the distance between where you are now and where you want to be is shorter than you think, so you need to find ways to keep your head in the right place until you get where you're trying to go.

Where does this continuous happiness and motivation come from? It comes from that place deep inside of you that refuses to accept the status quo. That place that knows that you *have* to keep going because living a life with so many limitations will never be an option for you.

I think of it like being lost in a forest. Imagine you've been walking for days. Or months. Or maybe even years. Understandably you're tired, and sometimes you even think about giving up, because no matter how much you walk, it feels like you'll never get out of this bloody forest. But the reality is, the reality that you can't yet see, is that you're only just a few trees away from getting through — from finally finding your way out and being free. Even though you can't see it yet, you're so incredibly close and giving up now would be tragic.

Sometimes when you're struggling it can feel like you're never going to get out of your current predicament and that things will never change. But they can, and they do. In fact, the only constant in life is change. You *know* this to be true. So know that these struggles you are currently experiencing are likely temporary. The only way out of this is through it.

One day, this day in front of us, is all we ever really have to deal with. Just master today, do the best you can, and then keep doing that every day. Let the future worry about itself.

Because each day, when viewed by itself, is doable. When I really think about it, there has never been one day in my life that contained more than I could handle. Not the day my mom took her own life, not the day my marriage ended, and not my worst day with CFS. I'm still here, alive and breathing. And I know you can get through those days too.

All that stress from a negative mindset impacts our health, so the state of our mind is going to have a massive impact on our rate of recovery from chronic illness. As Dr. Dean Ornish and

Anne Ornish explain in their book *Undo It! How Simple Life-style Changes Can Reverse the Onset of Most Chronic Diseases*, when stress is chronic it can increase inflammation in your brain which can lead to depression affecting not only your emotional state, but your immune system as well. It can also have a harmful effect on the millions of cells in your microbiome, along with negatively affecting many other systems in your body.

The good news, as these authors explain, is that stress comes primarily from our reactions to what happens to us, not from the events themselves. It's the perception of stress that matters. If we build up an arsenal of habits and skills to help us better cope with stress, we can be much happier and healthier as a result.

Indeed, Ornish and Ornish highlight that studies have shown that spending one hour per day on stress management techniques causes significant improvements in chronic health issues. Spending one hour per day on stress management techniques might seem like a lot to ask, but to put this in perspective, the average person spends over five hours per day on their mobile devices, plus a significant amount of time watching television. We definitely seem to always find a way to make time for the things that matter to us. If we want to see serious results with our health, we need to put in serious effort in managing our emotional well-being.

I've definitely found that controlling what happens in my mind, at least for a small portion of my day, is an essential practice for maintaining my overall happiness. When you're sitting with your eyes closed it might seem like you're not doing very much, but in fact, you're doing something quite powerful. Researchers at Harvard found that meditation alone can change the expression of genes that regulate inflammation, cell death (apoptosis), and oxidative stress in only a few weeks. Studies have shown that after only eight weeks of meditating thirty minutes per day there are measurable increases in the hippocampus, the part of your brain responsible for memory.[1] And with all the memory issues that come hand-in-hand with CFS, anything that can work to reverse this issue is definitely worth the effort.

Ornish and Ornish teach us that with meditation you can also rewire your brain to see things more positively. With just a few minutes a day you can launch yourself into an upward spiral and become that *glass half full* person you've always wanted to be. You become more resilient and better equipped to deal with life's challenges. I've read books on meditation, attended classes, used mobile apps, and even consulted some Buddhist monks on this topic, and my biggest takeaway from all this has been that meditation is something that's best kept simple. You don't need to be an expert at it to benefit from it.

I've found that pairing smaller chunks of meditation with everyday activities makes the process both more enjoyable and more realistic to do consistently. There are a few areas of my life that meditation pairs with nicely. I frequently go for massages, and I've noticed that during my massages, despite my body being in a state of total relaxation, my mind is often going a million miles a minute. Sometimes I'd try to imagine what my thoughts would sound like to the massage therapist if they were somehow able to be broadcasted from a speaker during my massage session. I was pretty sure I would sound insane. Now, each time I get a massage and I notice my thoughts running wild, it's my cue for me to meditate. I have a full hour to devote to clearing my mind, and when I leave, both my body and mind feel refreshed.

Another signal to meditate is when you feel yourself getting stressed by any encounter of any kind. For instance, if you find yourself in a frustrating conversation with someone, take a few moments and concentrate on what's happening in your mind and body. Imagine all the anger and frustration as a dark light flowing from the top of your head down to the bottom of your feet, draining into the earth, and dissolving into the earth's core. Next, imagine a white light filling up your body in all the places the dark light used to be, leaving you emanating love and peace out of every single one of your pores. It's pretty tough to hold onto negativity when you're filled to the brim with feelings of love and kindness.

If you aren't meditating in some way already, finding the time for even just sixty seconds per day will serve your happiness goals well. Pretty much any idle time throughout the day can be a good opportunity to get in some meditation. Time spent in an elevator or an Uber or in the waiting room at the doctor's office can all be transformed into helpful and calming meditation sessions. When all the bits and pieces of various forms of meditation in your day are tallied up, you will end up with a decent amount, and this practice makes a world of difference for your sanity.

I'm no expert on how to meditate, but I can offer these pointers: I highly recommend using a guided meditation app on your phone. I often use one called Headspace, and I really enjoy the array of topics covered in the app's meditations such as finding happiness, building confidence, improving sleep, dealing with anger, and so on.

I also wouldn't get too caught up in technique. Any time spent in silent reflection will do you some good. It's ok if during meditation your thoughts run wild like a cat on catnip. That doesn't mean you're doing it wrong. There is no *wrong*. If your thoughts won't calm down, simply sit silently and observe them instead. Watch them, note them, and then let them float along their merry way.

Using regular meditation spaces can also be helpful. It doesn't have to be the same space every single time, but if you have a few spots that you start to associate with meditation, it can help you relax quicker and get more from your meditation time.

Last but not least, although most sources seem to advocate meditating in the seated position, when I was sick with CFS I did my meditation lying down. I didn't want to waste any precious energy, and since I often had to lie down to rest anyway, it became another good opportunity to get in some meditation.

My favorite time to meditate is right before I go to bed. Typically, when I get into bed each night, my mind inevitably starts racing and examining every moment of my day, while simultaneously stressing about what is potentially to come the next day. To take control of all this pointless chatter, when I first crawl into bed I start by taking about sixty seconds to briefly review my day. I briefly touch on each of the highlights, like a light ball gently bouncing off each moment from my day. I follow this up with a quick mental scan of my body where I start with my head and move down to my toes and relax my body and release any tension that I find.

After you've reviewed your day and relaxed your body, deal with that voice in your head that, despite your need for sleep, insists on talking non-stop. I find it helpful to think of this voice as coming from a sort of super chatty little sister that resides in my brain. When it's time to go to sleep, I picture her inside my head, curled up in a ball with a blanket, and I say goodnight to her. I am in charge, not her, so I make it clear that I decide when bedtime is.

The main point of this meditation is to remind yourself at the end of each day that you are in control of the chatter in your head, and not vice versa. And it gives you a chance to enjoy some silence and easily drift off to sleep.

Regardless of what's going on in our lives, once we've tamed the dragons that plague our thoughts, we need to find ways to flood our minds with positive thoughts. Sometimes it's easy to lose our focus or perspective on things, and I've found that there are definitely things you can do daily that'll help ensure your head stays where you need it to.

For instance, I have folders set up on my phone for each day of the week. Each morning, shortly after I get out of bed and as I sip my freshly made lemon water, I open the folder for that day and flip through what I've stored inside. These folders are filled with inspirational quotes and memes from Instagram and quotes I've saved from books. Basically, all the things that I've come across that have spoken to me in some way end up in these folders. Whether it's using a photo organization app on your phone, some folders in your cloud storage account, or some other method that you use to organize things, it's easy-peasy to get yourself set up for this sort of daily dose of inspiration. If you're looking for someplace to get started, check out my Instagram account @raelan.agle. Accounts like @msrachel-hollis, @happsters, @melrobbins, and @daily_inspira-tional_quote_ put out some really uplifting stuff too.

I'm also a big believer in seeking out laughter. Who doesn't feel better after having a good laugh? Funny television series and movies became staples in my life when I was recovering from CFS, and they remain so today. Watching videos of comedians performing, following funny Instagram accounts, and hanging out with your funny friends are all important strategies for improving your happiness and mindset.

It may seem absurd to say that you should find things to be grateful for when struggling with CFS, but remember CFS does not define you. I personally keep a gratitude list that I read every day, but I know people who take a couple minutes once they are in bed and about to drift off to sleep to think about what they are grateful for. I've even had a gratitude box in my home. Each day that something wonderful happens that I am grateful for or want to remember, I write it down on a slip of paper and put it in the box. Then, on New Year's Eve, I open the box and take out all the slips of paper and read everything that I chose to write down throughout the year. I honestly can't think of a better way to finish off the year. Whichever way you do it, expressing gratitude can help you gain some perspective about all the good that is going on in your life and keep you from fixating on the negative.

And don't limit yourself to thoughts of gratitude. One way to cultivate positive emotions is to do an act of service, big or small, every single day — without expecting anything in return. These acts can provide a buffer against stress and depression.[2] This could be something as simple as sending out some kind messages on social media to other chronic illness sufferers, or as big as volunteering with a community organization in need of support. These acts can actually bring you some big rewards. And how amazing that a part of your healing plan can actually help someone else out as well.

Last but not least, don't neglect to focus on and celebrate your own personal successes. While recovering from CFS, keep a written log of everything you accomplish, whether big or small — every step taken toward your goal. I've used both a paper notebook and an online journal and found that both work great. Having a written record of all that you've accomplished can help keep that motivation going during the times that you're struggling. On days where you can only manage a fifteen-minute workout, you'll look back on a time when being able to walk to the end of your street to get the mail was a big success, and suddenly you'll have a whole new appreciation for your time at the gym. It's all about having perspective, and this log will be a handy dose of it for you whenever it's needed. Once I really got my healing plan on track, I had so many things to include in this journal that it was hard to keep up with them all. That was a great problem to have.

Journaling is something you can do at almost any time and in any place you want. It's a free beautiful moment in your day where you can put everyone and everything else aside and focus on just you.

I journal every single day. I'm not always excited to get started, but I *always* feel better afterward. Sometimes it's one paragraph; sometimes it's five pages. But whatever it is, for the most part, I always start my day by getting down something. Years ago, I liked using a paper journal that I kept in my nightstand and wrote in faithfully each night before bed. These days I've gone digital and prefer to explore my thoughts in the morning over a cup of kombucha.

I find that writing about your struggles can be incredibly cathartic. It's a great way to get your frustrations out, and by writing about the tough times you can start to work through them and piece together what might be amplifying your struggles and holding you back. I recommend writing with the mindset that you'll never ever go back and read what you've written. This keeps you from scripting your thoughts or from filtering them in any way. While journaling, you're not trying to sound eloquent or entertaining. Just let it flow. This will allow you to look at your life and your behavior a bit more honestly and help you be better able to sort through your struggles and figure out how to best handle them. If you choose to go back and read these journals later on, that's of course completely fine. And if you do, you'll appreciate the unfiltered candor with which you originally wrote them.

In addition to working through our daily struggles, it's essential to explore our past wounds as well. We all have them. Some of us are fortunate and have fewer than others, but no one gets through this life completely unscathed.

It's easy to tell ourselves that the past is in the past and is not really affecting us today in any significant way. I certainly thought that for most of my adult life. But I wasn't being honest with myself, because there were, in fact, quite a few things from my past that I still thought about a lot. Whether I wanted to admit it or not, as a result of certain events in my life I was holding onto feelings of frustration, guilt, shame, and inadequacy that continued to affect my behavior and my relationships with others.

When I decided to finally get serious about sorting through all of this, I started by making a list of everything I could think of from my past that still bothered me. And as it turned out, I actually had quite the laundry list of things persistently brewing below the surface. This list included virtually everything from my troubled teenage years, my failed marriage and other past relationships, my past financial irresponsibility, my issues with substance abuse, my ongoing fears about aging, my mother's illness and suicide, my own health issues and my

lack of independence, my toxic quest for perfec-
ly need to please others — just to name the big ones.

like a cliché examining my childhood to fix my
presc..., but it definitely worked. It turns out that this was a
pretty scary load to be carrying around. And let me tell you,
working through each of these items was intense business. It
was emotionally draining to write about these things. Some
days I actually felt ill after I finished writing. But more often
than not I felt euphoric. And each time I put to bed once and
for all some issue from my past, I felt so much lighter afterward.

I also recommend using your journal to look at what
limiting beliefs you might have that could potentially be
stunting your progress. If you believe that no one ever fully
recovers from CFS, then you likely won't either. If you believe
yourself to be a healthy person who is on the trajectory toward
vibrant health, then you likely will be.

And don't hesitate to make a point to write about the good
stuff as well. Even when my CFS was at its worst, I made sure
to write about how much I was learning, about how far I'd
come, and about how many good things were coming my way
one day very soon. Writing about the good helps you keep your
focus positive and your motivation strong to continue slugging
away at this horrid illness. And when you write about the good
things, don't just make up meaningless things to put down on
paper. Truly feel them. The more you write about them, the
more you will believe in their existence.

16

HABITS FOR HAPPINESS

I wish I could tell you that once you purge your mind of negative thoughts that you're ready to move forward toward better habits. But our negative mindset, it turns out, isn't just a mindset. Even if we get rid of the thoughts that plague us and actively work on our mental happiness, it turns out that we probably have some bad mental habits that we need to address as well.

In his book *Awaken the Giant Within*, Tony Robbins talks about using what he calls "transformational vocabulary" to shape your experiences in life. He teaches us that changing the words we use is the simplest tool for immediately transforming the quality of our lives. By using a transformational vocabulary, we can instantly change how we feel about what is happening to us, making this an incredibly powerful tool.

For instance, if you're having a bit of a rough day and you tell anyone who will stop long enough to listen how *today is really kicking your ass*, chances are that you will feel completely overwhelmed for the entirety of the day. But if you instead choose to tell people that *today had a couple challenging moments*, then it all instantly feels so much easier for you to manage and control. Robbins explains that by changing your habitual vocabulary — the words you consistently use to describe emotions — you can change how you think, how you feel, and how you live. I've tried this tactic countless times, and I always feel better afterward. And I'm sure the people around me have a better time of it too when the vocabulary I use is much less negative and dramatic.

If I'm completely honest, when I complain — when I talk about things that I'm struggling with — it feels as if I've opened a release valve in my body that allows some of my pain and frustration to flow out. Sometimes, being able to share my challenges with people who care about me feels really, truly helpful. But I've also found that this is something that I have to be careful with because talking about my struggles can sometimes do more harm than good.

When I first left Canada to travel around Southeast Asia, I made a decision to not talk about my health problems at all with anyone that I met. Not a single sentence. Not ever. *Nada.* My health had been my focus for so long, and I needed a break from CFS feeling like it was the center of my universe.

For almost a year I managed to not mention CFS to anyone, and not only did this give me a much-needed break from fixating on my illness, it actually shaped and transformed my experiences in that year for the better. I got to stop feeling like being sick was the defining part of who I was as a person, and when I look back on that year of travel, I don't even really remember being sick. Of course I still was, but by simply not talking about it, the illness actually became a much smaller part of my experience and my identity.

It's ok to need to talk to someone about your struggles; there's absolutely nothing wrong with that. It's important to be able to verbally work through our challenges and get support from others as we need it. I'm not saying that you need to take an entire year off from mentioning CFS. Just be aware of how the nature and extent to which you are talking about your illness is impacting your experience, and make sure that you are not making it a habit. If we are complaining just because we want attention, there's probably a better way to achieve that goal. Take a moment to look at the reasons for your venting and also at its outcomes.

That outcomes part is important. You want to make sure that all the wonderful people in your life actually want to be around you, and if you are complaining all the time, even the most well-intentioned people might start finding excuses to spend less time with you. Being a support person to a chronically ill person can be a hard and draining job, and you don't want to completely exhaust these valuable emotional care-givers. As challenging as it is to be the person who is sick, it's also difficult being the person who constantly has to hear about it. Just think about how much time *you* would want to spend around someone who talked about their problems all the time. As much as the people in your life love you and want to be there for you, it can be incredibly draining for them to continually hear about all your ailments and struggles.

When I notice myself repeating and oversharing the negative details of my life, sometimes it's because I feel desperate for people to understand what I'm going through. Although a completely understandable desire, unless the person sitting across from me has gone through something similar themselves, they will probably never understand what it's like — and I will go blue in the face trying to get them to.

You don't need every loved one in your life to understand what every minute of your day is like. When times are especially tough, share your struggles with those closest to you and let them know you're doing it because you need some support. And if something new develops in your list of ailments, share that as well. But if nothing is new and you are just repeating yourself, then try — for your sake and theirs — to keep your complaints to yourself.

As much as possible, make what you share with people be about other aspects of your life aside from illness. Aim to listen more than you talk. It's incredibly rewarding to be able to be there for others despite your own struggles. We all want to feel valuable, and turning the focus outward is one great way of accomplishing that.

In his book *Walden on Wheels: On the Open Road from Debt to Freedom*, Ken Illgunas describes his long and difficult journey to get himself out of crippling student-loan debt. Despite his intense frustration with this overwhelming financial burden, Ken also admitted the following:

Part of me liked being in that position of submission, tied up in leather, willfully cowering beneath a ruthless whip-yielding Sallie Mae. Life is simpler when we feel controlled. When we tell ourselves that we are controlled, we can shift the responsibility of freeing ourselves onto that which controls us. When we do that, we don't have to bear the responsibility of our unhappiness or shoulder the burden of self-ownership. We don't have to do anything. And nothing will ever change.

Quite honestly there was never a time when I wouldn't have practically sold my soul to have CFS removed from my life. As far as I am concerned, this illness is a life-sucking monster that just takes and takes and takes. So for a long time it definitely never occurred to me that I might actually be somehow *gaining* something from this whole ordeal.

But after taking a good, honest look at my life with CFS, reluctantly I had to admit that, however small, there were actually some benefits to being ill. Despite all the struggles CFS brought, being sick meant that many aspects of my life were much simpler. The expectations placed on me, by both myself and others, were far fewer. After years of being an over-achiever and running myself into the ground, finally feeling that I had the permission I needed to rest and take care of myself felt pretty good.

And despite hating being sick, I realized I wasn't so excited to return to the rat race. Having CFS allowed me to finally have a break to stop and breathe. Would recovering from CFS mean that once again my life would become insanely busy and difficult to manage? With my new, more relaxed outlook on life, the thought of going back to that lifestyle was pretty scary.

Admitting these things to myself allowed some doubts to creep in. *Is it possible that on some level I actually don't want to get better?* Loathing CFS the way I did, it was a tough thing to think about. But I had to admit, there was a small part of me that thrived while being ill. It was only a small corner of my brain that relished the idea of keeping my break from the responsibilities of life going, but how much power did that small corner have? What sort of havoc was my mind wreaking? Was it somehow keeping me sick?

These are important questions that need to be addressed

repeatedly throughout your CFS journey to ensure you aren't, in fact, getting in your own way. You have to make sure you remove *all* incentives to remaining ill. Start using your recovery time to figure out what you want and need from life *once you get well*. Imagine a new and different healthy lifestyle for yourself, one in which you balance your obligations with self-care and don't need to contract a disease in order to get some rest. Think about all the ways you could be healthy, meet the demands of life, and still get the rest and relaxation time that you crave.

You also have to make sure that illness is not part of your identity, because once something becomes a part of who we think we are, it can be a tough thing to get rid of. If your Instagram handle is *@chronicallyillkathy,* you might want to take a long beat and consider what psychological impact this is having on your recovery process. It's important to keep illness separate from yourself, something you can easily put down and walk away from when your body is ready. You have to be clear in your mind that illness is serving no helpful purpose in your life and that 100 percent of your mind and body should be on board with eradicating it.

I've been talking about bad habits that we can get ourselves into and how to avoid them. Unfortunately, bad habits are not limited to just how we talk or how we see ourselves. Believe it or not (and I'm willing to bet you believe it), other people can be bad habits as well.

When you are learning how to care for yourself as you work on your recovery from CFS, you need to do only those things that keep yourself feeling emotionally good and strong. This needs to be as big a priority as all the other aspects of your healing plan. But it's not just about doing certain things — it's also about certain people. After spending time with the various people in your life, pay attention to how you feel. Do you feel uplifted, inspired, supported, and energized? Or do you feel drained and even more exhausted than before you spent time with them? If it's the latter, you should strongly consider limiting your contact with them until you have the emotional resources to handle the negativity that they bring to the relationship.

The same thing goes for the activities and situations to which you expose yourself. If that mindfulness meditation always leaves you feeling frustrated, it has to go. If that kundalini yoga class that has helped every single person you know to thrive in life always leaves you feeling frustrated and drained, ditch it. If that one awesomely organic café your friend always wants to meet at is so loud that you can't find the energy to think while you're there, go someplace else.

Now life would be simple if you could just walk away from someone or someplace that is a drain on your energy. But what do you do with that experience — the memory of what happened? That can eat you alive just as much as being in the presence of that person or in that place.

In the last chapter I talked about how judgment and negative emotions can sabotage us. Well, I'm here to tell you that they can do the same thing when we try to deal with the people around us as well. When someone is behaving in a way that makes us unhappy, it's easy to get angry and to start judging them. All sorts of questions and frustrations can start going through our minds and clouding our ability to deal with the situation effectively.

When I feel my blood starting to boil, I like to mentally throw that person into an imaginary observation room in my mind. It's like the soundproof interrogation rooms on TV, where I can observe that person's behavior while I'm safely behind a one-way mirror, and I can choose whether to hear what they're saying. Once I safely store the annoying person in that room in my mind, I let them do their thing for a bit while I calm myself down.

From this safe distance, I'm now free to observe what's happening with that person or situation. It doesn't usually take long for me to conclude that the rantings of this person I've placed in this sealed room are mostly about them and have very little to do with me. What felt like a personal assault in fact probably wasn't personal at all. Despite not being able to control their behavior, I have the ability to control my own. Their behavior is all about them, and how I react is all about me.

This goes to my larger point about taking care of your emotions. It's ok to feel like a mess for a little while, because all of this self-care is your path to clarity and your way out of the mess you're in. But because you are feeling what you're feeling, I want to give you permission to say no to as many things as possible, because right now it needs to be all about you.

Let me be clear: this isn't being selfish. It really is challenging to be good for anyone else when you are struggling with CFS, so even though your healing journey should be primarily about you, it is very much for the sake of the other people in your life as well. It's almost impossible to be a good mother, father, partner, friend, child, or employee if you yourself are not in a good place. We are pretty much useless to others when we don't take care of ourselves.

This healing plan isn't going to work unless you do, so if you want to get better, you need to truly focus on that and make it your absolute priority. Invest this time in yourself now so that you can have many great years to come where you can fully enjoy this world and all the people in it. Once you are better, you can go back to being there for others. For now, you need to make *you* priority number one. The world will keep turning, I promise.

───────────

Just so we're clear, I'm not saying you should cut off contact with other people and isolate yourself. In fact, just the opposite. During those early years with CFS, when I was mostly housebound, I felt pretty isolated. Some days I actually resorted to refreshing the weather page on my computer just to feel some sort of connection to the world. It sounds ridiculous and oh so sad, but it actually really did help just a little bit. I needed to feel some sort of connection to the world around me, even if just for a minute.

If connecting with the online weather network can help a person feel less alone, imagine what connecting with an actual human can do for our well-being. Actually, you don't have to imagine it. The research is clear: love, happiness, and meaningful connections with others enhance health. Research has shown that people who feel loved and supported are much more likely to make and maintain lifestyle choices that are life-enhancing. People who feel lonely, depressed, and isolated are three to ten times more likely to get sick and die prematurely from virtually all causes when compared to those who have strong feelings of love, connection, and community.[1]

I know that when you're suffering from serious chronic fatigue, maintaining any sort of social life can feel next to impossible. I get that; I really do. But I've learned that even though it might not be the easiest thing to do while sick, it's so important to try to keep your key friendships alive. You've likely spent years building up many of these relationships, and to let them go now would be terrible. Your key people, your tribe, will be super happy to come over to your home once in a while, have a cup of tea, and just visit with you for a bit. For the same reasons that you keep them in your life, they keep you in theirs as well. They like you! I'm sure you've been there for them in the past when they needed it and will continue to enthusiastically show up to have their backs in the future when you are recovered and you are able. And when you're struggling, they'll want to be able to be there for you and support you. In fact, they might be offended if they later learn how much you were struggling and that you never once reached out to them for support.

Right now is your turn to be on the receiving end of all that love and compassion. Don't be afraid to reach out and ask for what you need from people, because spending time in person with a friend or family member that you cherish can be absolutely magical. People aren't mind readers. They don't know what you want, need, or expect from them. They might assume that since you've turned down their last seventeen dinner invitations (and bless their souls for, despite your repeated refusals, continuing to invite you), you are just too sick to visit. Let people know what works for you and what you currently *can* still do.

Ever since I've had the option, I've been an avid, shameless user of social media. I'm not suggesting it should be a complete replacement for face-to-face human contact, but it can definitely be a great supplement.

These days, there is an online group out there for virtually everything imaginable. If you aren't already connected to this wonderful world of support and information, it's time to get started. During tough times, connection with others who understand what you are going through is so incredibly important. Find groups that discuss things that you care about and are filled with people who are going through what you are going through. Don't just *like* posts, but share your comments, send private messages, and just generally get engaged in the conversations that are happening. Trust me, as long as you are coming from a place of love, the people on the receiving end will cherish the thoughts and feedback you give.

But just as with face to face interactions, being surrounded online by chronic complainers is not good for your health or happiness. Use fierce boundaries with your online content. Unfollow or "hide" accounts from those people whose posts don't uplift you. Keep your online space sacred and filled with only uplifting people and content. Everyone's allowed to have a bad day and do a teeny bit of venting online, but if this is their pattern then they have to go.

When it comes to improving my face-to-face relationships, social media, for me, is actually pure gold. The people who are in my life are there for a reason. It's because I adore and cherish them and having this online opportunity to keep up with them in some capacity, all while sipping my almond milk iced latte and lounging at home on my couch is such an incredible thing. And it means that when I do get to have my next cherished face-to-face meeting with them, since I already know that their seven-year-old won a silver medal at their latest dance competition, or that they just had the most amazing of holidays in Italy, we can pick up where we left off so much quicker. With social media I feel more integrated into people's lives which, for me, is incredibly important.

I have a final recommendation for you, one I think you should seriously consider: see a professional counselor. I'd go to counseling on a full-time basis for the rest of my life if my budget allowed for it. No joke. It's not because I think I'm so incredibly messed up. It's because I firmly believe that, no matter what's happening in your life, counseling can always help you make things even better.

Like anything else, you might have to shop around for a bit before you find a counselor who's a good fit for you. It might all feel a little annoying in the beginning and like a total waste of your time, energy, and money. But it's not. Because the support you receive from a professional counselor is not something that can be duplicated through friends and family. With a counselor, you get to focus 100 percent on yourself, with no worry about how much you're unloading on that person. Unload away! That is *exactly* what they are there for. They are there to focus on you. To support you. To help you figure out your life and how to live the best version of it possible. It's a beautiful thing, really, and it's unfortunate that more people aren't willing or able to take advantage of this massive opportunity for growth.

Whatever it looks like, find something that works for you, and get connected with some people around you. Emotional support is absolutely a vital part of your healing plan. You need that beautiful connection with others to get well, so don't neglect this important part of your recovery.

VII

AT LIBERTY TO LIVE

17

THE MYTH OF WILLPOWER

One summer day, years before I got CFS, I was out shopping at my favorite local mall and looking for a new bikini to buy. As I walked through one of the swimsuit stores I excitedly collected a handful of bikinis to try on. They all looked so cool on the rack, and I was so excited to see which one would be the perfect fit for my upcoming lake trip with friends. One after another I tried them all on and discovered that every single one looked horrendous on me.

Despite how much I went to the gym at the time, I was still in the throes of my sugar addiction, so I yo yo-ed with my weight and struggled to keep off those extra few pounds that stubbornly clung to my midsection. These swimsuits that looked so cute on the rack highlighted my seemingly endless unwanted bulges and ripples. I couldn't imagine wearing a single one of them out in public. It was devastating. I remember standing in that tiny change room with those dreadful fluorescent lights and feeling so depressed about the state of my body. I left the store frustrated and empty-handed.

After I left the store I walked around the mall in a bit of a daze. I felt like a failure and was feeling pretty hopeless that I'd ever be able to attain a body that I was truly proud of. While on this walk of self-pity I passed a bakery that oozed the intoxicating scent of chocolate and had on display some of the most delectable-looking chocolate chip cookies I'd ever seen. So in an effort to cheer myself up and try to pull myself out of this slump, I bought myself a treat to eat as I continued on with my shopping.

As I ate my giant cookies, I found that I felt better from the sugar high, but also worse from the shame of it all. I was somehow attempting to use my problem (my sugar consumption) as the solution to this day's disaster (not looking good in a bikini), and it was all just so ridiculous. I was better than this! I thought of myself as a strong person and couldn't understand why I couldn't stick to a simple plan that, if followed, would get me exactly what I wanted. All I had to do was eat healthily and be active, and I would look and feel great. Why did that feel so impossible to achieve?

I used to think of willpower as some elusive mystical quality that people either had or they didn't. If they had it, we're not sure how they got it, or where exactly it came from. It's apparently something that just appears for them, as if by magic, whenever needed.

Though rarely shown how to cultivate this same quality in ourselves, we're taught to admire these strong people and marvel at their apparently innate ability to use their ever-present willpower to make such exceptional choices in their lives. When the time comes for us to require some of this amazing strength to overcome some personal hurdle, we tell ourselves we can't do it. That we're not strong enough. That we're just not built like those other people. That for us, it's just too hard.

Fortunately, I've since learned that none of this is true. And thank the stars for that, because how horribly unfair and frustrating would it be if some of us were just born weak.

Recovering from CFS can seem really hard and overwhelming and at times on the verge of impossible. It can be scary, which can make it all too easy to start doubting ourselves and our abilities to make it all happen. Sometimes it feels like we are too weak. Like we aren't cut out for this. Like there's no way we can muster the strength to do what's needed to make ourselves well again.

In my quest to conquer CFS, I've discovered that the concepts of willpower and strength thankfully are myths — or at the very least they're not what we conventionally believe them to be. We've decided that strength and willpower are what get successful people where they are, when in fact these traits on their own rarely get anyone anywhere.

In his book *Willpower Doesn't Work — Discover the Hidden Keys to Success*, psychologist Benjamin Hardy, PhD, drives home the fact that we cannot rely on willpower because we can only use it for a limited amount of time before it inevitably gives out. Hardy insists that relying on willpower will, without a doubt, lead to failure because it just won't last if our environment is in conflict with our goals. It doesn't matter how *strong* you are — eventually, the environment always wins.

Strength is just a word we use to describe what people see when we make a specific type of choice. It's choosing to do the right thing over the wrong thing, choosing good over bad. When we remove the word *strength* from any situation and instead look at things as choices to be made, we see that we are the ones in control. If we make a healthy, desirable decision, people say we are strong. If we make an unhealthy decision, people say we are weak.

So setting aside the language of strong and weak, the question really is just how do we make sure that we can easily make the right choices in life and avoid the wrong ones? If it's not strength or willpower, then what is it? And how do we make sure we always know what the right decision is?

Since we have to make countless decisions each and every day, it's just not realistic to think that we can properly evaluate every situation that comes along to see what course of action is best. *Will I get more joy or benefit from eating or not eating that piece of cake? Taking the elevator or the stairs? Being friendly to my neighbor or putting my head down and pretending I don't see him?* With all of these decisions thrown at us all day long we can't possibly make the decisions that are best for us each and every time. Conducting a thorough cost-benefit analysis for each and every decision that we have to make just isn't realistic. And if we are relying on willpower to make the best decisions, then we are really in trouble.

Since we can't rely on willpower or on having the time and motivation to repeatedly make the best decisions for ourselves all day long, we need to look at what happens when we make good and bad decisions and figure out how to structure our environments and our minds so that we have more of the good factors and fewer of the bad.

Sometimes it can feel like we keep making the wrong decisions, decisions that are not at all in line with our goals, but for some reason, we keep making them anyway. This can leave us feeling like failures. If you find yourself in this pattern, it's not weakness or lack of willpower that's holding you back. You might have chalked it up to this, but thankfully the reality is that it's something much more concrete and much more fixable.

If I believe that a choice I'm making will, without a doubt, do me some good and bring me happiness, I will easily make that choice. Every time. All day. Every day. If someone I trust offers me some free money, I take it. It's a no-brainer. I believe to my core that money makes my life easier and better so I will always happily accept some when it comes my way.

If someone were to offer me a glass of drain cleaner to drink, I could quickly and easily turn it down. By saying *no* to the poisonous beverage, I get to avoid drinking something that likely tastes disgusting, and I will also most likely get to live to see another day.

Now let's say that I keep saying yes to offers of deep-fried chocolate-covered bacon. Even though I might say to myself and others that I know this kind of snack is not good for me and that I plan to stop eating it, I keep eating it anyway. And after I eat it, I berate myself for being weak and giving in to things I said I should avoid.

One reason I might keep eating junk food despite continuous vows to stop is because I don't completely believe that this behavior is doing me that much harm. After all, there's a healthy and fit looking person standing next to me eating the same snack, and they are clearly doing fine. We use the *everybody does it* defense, as if that somehow magically makes it not harmful for us. If I haven't totally bought into all the reasons that I should stop this behavior, I likely won't stop. Once I understand and believe with every fiber of my being that this behavior is doing me more harm than good, I will stop.

Humans are selfish creatures, so we basically only do things that benefit us. If I give to charity, it's likely because I feel better about myself as a person afterward and it lessens the guilt I experience about the messed-up state of the world. If I leave my boyfriend a nice note on his bathroom mirror, on some level I know that he will likely also then do nice things for me and that our relationship overall will be better as a result. We humans like to think of ourselves as capable of selfless acts, but when you break it down, it's pretty hard to make a convincing argument that we are.

If we choose to have a giant piece of chocolate cake, it's partly because on some level (regardless of what we tell ourselves and others) we believe that having that cake will bring more joy to our lives than abstaining from it will. We don't really think that it's all that bad. We haven't fully bought into the benefits that abstaining from cake-eating, so we indulge. Once we completely internalize and fully believe all the ways we will suffer as a result of eating too much cake, we will happily and easily leave it untouched. If we can't seem to leave the cake alone, then we probably don't believe that the sacrifice of not eating it is worth the reward for abstaining.

If you find you are struggling with your decision-making in a specific area, try educating yourself more about the topic. If you want to stop eating processed meats, watch some documentaries or read some books that detail their harmful effects. Do some trial runs on healthier diets and document how you feel while eating them. Ignorance is the enemy here. Once you educate yourself and fully understand how much happiness a certain behavior is stealing from you, you'll leave it behind.

Another reason we might be making bad choices is because we have become masters at lying to ourselves. We might focus on that one random study we heard about telling us that to be healthy we should drink alcohol every day, while we ignore the countless other studies that detail the endless toxic effects of regular alcohol consumption. We put our heads in the sand and simply refuse to hear any new information that doesn't support our bad habits. Or we just straight-up lie to ourselves about the nature of our behavior. We tell ourselves we can have a piece of chocolate cake because we rarely ever have any, when in reality we actually eat sugary treats almost every single day. We lie to ourselves and pretend we have our problematic behaviors under control, when in fact these behaviors are in control of us.

In short, we pretend everything is ok, when it is anything but.

These days, it's easier than ever to remain in denial about our unhealthy habits. We have almost completely normalized our sedentary, junk food-fueled lives to the point where this absurdly toxic behavior requires almost no explanation or justification at all.

If two friends go to a party, and one sucks back gin and tonics all night long while the other sticks to water, which one do you think will be more likely have to explain themselves to others before the night is through? What about that guy in your office cafeteria who eats a lot of salad, brings his own dressing, and weighs his food, compared to the guy who sits next to him eating bacon double-cheeseburgers with an extra-large Coke every single day? Who will likely have to justify their behavior to others more often? It's ironic and a bit frustrating that often those people who are making smart and healthy choices are the ones that find that they have a lot of explaining to do.

If there is a certain situation that every time it comes up you keep making the "wrong" decision, take a moment to take a look at what you are really telling yourself about this behavior. What lies are you telling yourself? What information are you ignoring? Have you done the research but are pretending that it supports your bad habits? Are you lying to yourself about how often you do something or the extent to which it has control over you? The incredible thing is that once we shine a light on our denial, it makes it impossible for that denial to continue to work. Once we pull our head out of the sand, it's really hard to put it back in. Once we've recognized the ways in which we've tricked and fooled ourselves, there's no going back. A good, honest assessment of our thoughts and beliefs about a certain behavior can be a total game-changer.

Other times when we think we make too many bad decisions, we actually just have an accumulation of bad habits.

There's no getting around it; we all have a ton of habits. The good news is that it's up to us to decide whether we are victims or beneficiaries of these habits.

Habit is just another word for a specific decision in your life that's been automated. To ensure my life is as easy and productive as possible, I aim to automate as many decisions as I can. Once I've figured out how I want to act in a specific recurring situation, I commit to always acting that way and never make a decision about it again. I turn that one decision about that one situation into a rule, ensuring I never have to think about what to do in that scenario ever again. And just like that, a habit is born. Over time that habit will strengthen and become such an ingrained part of my life that I'll barely even register what's happening. If it's a good habit, this can be a really powerful thing.

For instance, let's take a look at one of my old nemeses: sugar. Perhaps after I've learned how bad it is for my body, I've decided that I don't want to eat too much refined sugar, but that I also don't want to be overly rigid with myself and remove it entirely. This leaves an almost endless array of situations in which I'll still have to decide whether or not to eat sugar. But I'm going to have a meltdown if I have to make a decision in each and every instance.

To remedy this, I take a moment and make a rule that serves to automate my behavior whenever I encounter sugar. The rule doesn't have to be complicated to be effective. In fact, the simpler the better. I could decide that my rule for sugar is that I'll eat it only on weekends and never in my own home. This rule is simple, clear, and it covers virtually every possible situation I'll ever encounter. If I'm at work and a coworker brings in a batch of sugary baked goods, assuming I have a Monday-to-Friday job, I know without even having to think about it that I won't have any, because I don't eat sweet treats during the week. When I'm grocery shopping and am bombarded with aisles and aisles of sugar-filled items, I no longer need to muster up that magical willpower to abstain from buying them. Since I'll be bringing these groceries to my home, a place where no added sugar is consumed, I know that I will not be buying anything. If, on the other hand, I'm at a party at a friend's house on a Saturday night, without any thought or internal debate, I know that if I want some, I can have a piece of her birthday cake.

With this one small automation of my behavior I've removed decision-making from so many areas of my life, thus eliminating the need to time and time again find that mythical strength and willpower needed to stay on track. I make the decision one time and then move on with my life. And the more I do it, the more ingrained it becomes. By automating my behavior, that exhausting and repetitive internal struggle is gone. It's the difference between a one-off choice and a lifestyle change. And the more I start automating behaviors, the more I want to do it. When I see the benefits of automation, it makes me want to remove the decision-making step from as many areas of my life as possible.

In his book *Atomic Habits: An Easy & Proven Way to Build Good Habits & Break Bad Ones*, author James Clear describes the power of accumulating small positive habits over time. Clear calls small habits the "compound interest of self-improvement" because, in the beginning, it's hard to see how these small contributions are really getting us anywhere in the long run. But just as with compound interest, when we master multiple tiny behaviors in our lives, we eventually see remarkable results.

When making changes to improve your health, it can be frustrating to see how little change is happening in the first days, weeks, and months, and it might not seem like you're getting anywhere. Clear explains that to see the benefits of small behavior changes, we need to focus on our current trajectory rather than our current results. He suggests imagining shifting the route of an airplane by just a few degrees. Initially this might not seem like a big change, but in reality, this change could result in the plane landing in an entirely different country than where it was initially headed.

Clear also points out that, in the same way that tiny behavior changes can result in incredible progress, they can also result in massive deterioration in our lives. Duplicating small mistakes day after day will have the same compound effect. Our accumulation of small choices, if they are the wrong ones, will have toxic results. So as much as we need to pay attention to where our behaviors are getting us, we need to look at where they *aren't* getting us as well.

Clear points out that winners and losers have the same

goals. For the most part, everyone wants to achieve happiness, success, health, and financial stability. So it's not our goals that define whether we will be successful or not. He maintains that you need to focus less on the goals and more on the systems that will get you there. Even though it's hard to recognize, the glory is to be found in the small, everyday things that you do.

To the outside world, much of what people accomplish ends up looking like an overnight success. But the reality is most of us only broadcast the positive end results. I don't have pictures of myself with CFS lying sick in bed day after day, but I sure as heck have pictures of myself thriving in life once I got well. And until we are successful, no one is paying much attention to what we broadcast anyway. But it's all the work that's done in the beginning when it seems like we aren't making any progress that makes the end result possible. Your success will be the product of good daily habits. It isn't a one-time transformation.

When it comes to changing your habits when suffering from CFS, I believe that starting slow with small changes is the best approach to take. I had to learn to override my love of jumping into things headfirst and appreciate how to take things more slowly instead. Precious energy stores can be depleted if you try and make too many changes all at once. When setting your goals, commit to making some small changes first and then build on those as your energy levels allow.

James Clear explains what he calls the "Two Minute Rule." This rule states that when you start a new habit it should take less than two minutes to do. If you want to start journaling daily, start by writing only a couple sentences per day. If you want to start a regular meditation practice, start with two minutes per day. The idea is to make your habits as easy as possible to start. A new habit should not feel like a challenge. A daily two-minute walk can eventually grow to a daily thirty-minute walk. When the first two minutes of any habit is easy, it becomes a gateway habit that will eventually lead you down a more productive path.

The point, according to Clear, is to master the habit of showing up, because a habit must be established before it can be improved. You can't make any significant progress if you can't master the simple habit of being present. Very few people can master a near-perfect habit from the start. You have to standardize before you can optimize.

It's important to know when to call it quits on a habit too. I feel a bit like a failure every time I try something and then have to abandon it. Sometimes I want to stick with the habit, despite the fact that it's not actually getting me anywhere, just so I can say I followed through on my plans. The identity of being someone who follows through on things is very important to me, and few things give me more satisfaction in life than having a plan and sticking to it to the letter. But sometimes a plan that sounds good in theory doesn't actually help me, and it's important to recognize this quickly so that I can drop this strategy and replace it with a better one.

Speaking of identifying as a person who follows through — sometimes what feels like a lack of willpower is actually just a problematic identity that we've adopted. This can happen when we've internalized our poor decision-making to the point where it's become a part of who we think we are. If laziness is something that you think you experience only on occasion, then this belief likely won't hold you back too much if you decide to live a more active lifestyle. But if you think that being lazy is *who you are*, then you're likely prone to make decisions in your life that support that identity.

Clear insists that changing behaviors isn't only about the accumulation of small productive habits, but it's an identity change as well. He explains that a really effective way to ensure you are on board with the small behaviors that you're trying to cultivate in your life is to make them a part of your identity. Decide that you, as a person, are someone who does not eat junk food. Be proud of who you are and how you live your life in this healthy way. Once your pride gets involved, you'll fight tooth-and-nail to maintain your habits. Clear explains that you must begin acting like the type of person you already know yourself to be, and think carefully about what kind of person that is.

If you are a person suffering from CFS, don't think of yourself as a sick person trying to get well; your actions and habits identify you as *a healthy person who is removing CFS from your life*. Healthy people experience sickness, and this is just one of those experiences. You eat well, you exercise as much as is healthy for your body at this time, and you learn as much as you can about health and healing. That, by my definition, is a healthy person. Take pride in that and live that way each and every day.

We all live within the limits of our current situation. The average person cannot just get up one morning and decide to run a marathon. You have to start small, train, and work your way up to that. But throughout that training process, even before ever having successfully completed a marathon, that person likely thinks of themselves as a runner. Once it becomes an integral part of who you are, you will do whatever is needed to make sure your actions are in line with that identity.

But as with habits, the power of identity is a double-edged

sword. If you believe yourself to be someone who isn't active, who is unhealthy, or who doesn't eat well, you'll emulate the behaviors of that identity. Clear insists that you need to decide who you want to be and prove to yourself that you are that person with small wins as you go.

The real reason habits matter is because they change your beliefs about yourself. You don't need to be perfect. Look at the average of your behavior-change over time. Your chart might not show a flawless diagonal line going up toward your goal. The line will likely be jagged, with some days being better than others. But over time you will make fewer errors, and you will fine-tune your behavior with each passing day. As long as the overall trajectory is up, you are headed in the right direction — and that is what you should be paying attention to.

Sometimes what feels like weakness is actually just us putting ourselves in the wrong environment. If I'm trying to cut out dessert, then going to the restaurant that always has my favorite cake on display isn't going to make this very easy for me. If I want to stop drinking, then hanging out in bars probably isn't the best idea. If I know I need a quiet environment to get some writing done on my book, then hanging out in loud and busy coffee shops probably isn't going to get me anywhere.

It's such a simple thing, but by putting ourselves in the right environment we are much more likely to make the right decisions that support our goals. If my goal is to eat a healthy brunch on Sunday, then I'll suggest to my friends that we go try that new organic vegan café I just saw advertised. If I want to hang out with creative and healthy people, then I'll go to art and yoga classes to make friends. If I'm struggling to stick to my budget, I'll hang out at a park instead of a shopping mall in my spare time.

Avoiding problematic environments isn't a sign of weakness but rather the opposite. Making conscious decisions about how and where to spend your time is an admirable quality in anyone. Set yourself up for success by filling your environment with the people and things that move you closer toward your goals.

But environments are not just passive places — they can and should be actively shaped by you. It's not just where we go that impacts our success, but also what we place or don't place in those environments that shapes our behavior.[1] If you want to go to the gym more often, leave your gym shoes out and gym bag by the front door. Hang a calendar on your wall in a room you spend a lot of time in, and mark a huge green checkmark on it for each day you go to the gym. Put healthy snacks in the most visible and easily accessed places in your kitchen, and keep a water bottle on your desk so that you'll drink healthy beverages instead of sugary ones. Use a picture of a desired holiday destination as wallpaper on your phone or computer to motivate you to stick to your health recovery plan and to keep working on getting strong enough to go there. Invite friends over to visit who you know won't bring junk food or want a beer when they arrive. Make plans with your friends for lunch instead of dinner if you think that will make you less likely to consume alcohol. Clear emphasizes that, whatever you do, you should work to shape your environment to have as many positive cues as possible so that it will be easy to stick to your plan and achieve your goals.

Trying to white-knuckle our way through change might work in the short run, but in the long run, this is almost never a successful strategy. If we want to be someone who is strong, meaning that we want to be that person who does all the right things every day that will bring us the best possible results, then we need to take a close look at these various dimensions of strength and see if all are in order in our lives. Because it's not actually strength or willpower that will get you where you want to go — it's information, awareness, planning, and skills.

We all have habits that are running our lives, or we live in denial. Our lack of buy-in is directly related to the harmful environments we find ourselves in. We need to examine our mental programming and take stock of what beliefs are taking us toward our goals and which ones are taking us further away. We chalk up so much of achieving results to motivation, but motivation is overrated. Having a plan is more important. By having a plan you remove the tendency to fall into old habits and instead create a new identity: a healthier, habitually happier you.

18

PRACTICE MAKES PERFECT

Once you understand that willpower is a myth, you can carry that belief over into different practical aspects of your life. I want to share with you some concrete examples of how I liberated myself from the tyranny of thinking that I lacked willpower.

For the longest time, having a comprehensive list detailing every single thing that I needed to get done felt to me like the backbone of a productive and efficient life. There was a time where I probably had lists that were just lists of other lists that I needed to make. I. Loved. Lists.

Oh, the hours I've spent making, organizing, and pouring over my To-Do lists. They had an inexplicable yet undeniable power over me. I checked my lists compulsively. If I didn't look at my lists multiple times a day, I'd have this constant feeling of fear and anxiety that I was somehow forgetting something really important.

Sure, these lists did generally help me get things done, but the less desirable items always got pushed to the end, meaning that some items always took ages to complete. With a To-Do list, it's just too easy to procrastinate on some items and never really get to them. As long as I was crossing some items off the list each day, I felt productive and on top of my life. This system made it easy to ignore the times when I was avoiding all the tough stuff and really just concerning myself with being able to cross some stuff off.

Worst of all was that I never had a single day where everything on that list was completed — a day where I was ever truly free of outstanding chores. I always had obligations and unfinished tasks hanging over my head and stealing my happiness from any downtime I might take. I never really had any guilt-free spare time. There was always something to be done, always something waiting for me.

In other words, I thought I lacked the willpower to complete my lists.

Thankfully, I've found another way to live — a better way that is completely free of To-Do lists and any lingering guilt that somehow I lack willpower. Now instead of making lists, I make choices: I have a **schedule**.

I replaced my lists with a **calendar** that tells me only what I need to do for that day and nothing else. When something comes up in life that I previously would've put on my To-Do list, I now assign that task to a specific date on my calendar. This way I can relax and forget about it completely until the day I've decided that it will get done. I no longer have to look at that item every single day on some list and try to decide if today is the day I will finally do it. And on the very rare occasion that a reminder comes up on my calendar for something and I find that I can't get it done on that day, I **reschedule** it for another specific date in the future and do it then.

When it comes to organizing my time, here's exactly how I do it: I start off each morning in a note-taking app called Evernote, where I put together a schedule for that day. It's a simple schedule where I simply list some times down the left side of the page, with each task that needs to be completed that day plugged into a specific time slot.

I consult two sources that tell me what my tasks are for the day. The first is my digital calendar, which might contain items such as doctor's appointments, picking up dry cleaning, etc. I see at what times each of these things needs to happen and put them in my schedule for the day in my Evernote app.

The second source I consult to see what tasks need to be completed is a weekly chart I've made up that has all the tasks and items such as cleaning and laundry that reoccur every single week on certain days. Having this second chart of basic, weekly repeating tasks keeps my digital calendar from getting too bogged down and makes it easy to spot important items on the calendar at a glance.

To make this weekly chart, I started off by making a list of all the things that need to get done each and every week. This might include items such as laundry, ironing, house cleaning, exercise time, watering the plants, doing meal planning, getting groceries, doing meal preparation, reviewing my finances, and even getting massages. Then I take the simple weekly chart that I've made and list each task under the heading of a certain day. For example, laundry gets assigned to Monday, watering the plants to Thursday, groceries to Saturday, and so on. I keep this weekly master chart at the bottom of the Evernote page I use to create my daily schedule, so all I have to do is scroll down to see what's there.

By reducing my life to just these two calendars I've simplified my life greatly. It might sound a bit complicated, but it's really not. While having my morning tea I simply open up

Evernote, look at my weekly master chart and my digital calendar and see what items are there, and plug those items into a schedule for that day. (If you'd rather have everything in just the one place, using a calendar for everything works fine too.)

Below is an example of what my Monday schedule would look like after plugging the tasks in from my weekly master chart (a snippet of which I've included below as well):

Making a daily schedule is important for a couple reasons. For one, without the schedule, you will probably just end up making a To-Do list for the day — and we already know all the hassles and annoyances that these kinds of lists bring. You'll leave the least desirable items for last, some items might never get done, and all day long you'll have stuff hanging over you and robbing you of your peace. Also, without a schedule, it's almost impossible to figure out how and when you will fit everything in.

Another reason why a daily schedule is important is that, by eliminating lists and scheduling instead, I free up my mind and energy for other things. I can either spend my life repeatedly looking down at my overgrown, chipped fingernails, feeling guilty about not taking care of them and wondering when I'll get to them, or I can plug this task into my calendar. Because when I always know there is time devoted to taking care of them, I never have to criticize myself about my nails again. It's incredible how freeing such a simple practice can be.

THURS	FRI	SAT	SUN
•organize day plan	•organize day plan	•organize day plan	•organize day plan
•journal	•journal	•journal	•journal
•write/work	•write/work	•CFS social media	•CFS social media
•CFS social media	•CFS social media	•workout	•clean house
•plan weekend	•workout	•groceries	•meal prep
•review budget	•make next week's	•manicure & pedicure	•water plants
•meditate	meal plan & grocery list	•meditate	•get massage
•learn/watch	•meditate		•meditate
educational videos	•learn/watch		
	educational videos		

As my day goes along, sometimes I'll need to tweak my schedule and adjust the times as I go. As long as I am legitimately attempting to follow it and doing my best to stay on track, I don't stress at all about minor changes. After all, my calendar is there to keep me on track, and if I've overbooked myself, I just reschedule.

One last thing I do to manage my schedule is to put a reminder on my calendar on the first of January each year to plug in all the repeating monthly and yearly tasks I have. On my Evernote page with my daily and weekly schedule, I also have a yearly master list of items that require attention. At the start of each new year, I take this list and plug the items into my calendar for the year. Some of them are always on the same date (such as birthdays, anniversaries, and filing taxes), so I can set a repeating reminder and never have to worry about them again. Other items that aren't always on the same date (such as times slotted for periodic budget reviews, juice cleanses, organizing my photos, etc.) I need to manually plug into my calendar each year. Once all these tasks are slotted in for the year, I can forget about all of these things and not waste another moment worrying about them.

If you want to free up significant time and energy, ditch the To-Do list. Put everything on a schedule so you don't have to think about it. Schedule all tasks and then forget them until they pop up on your calendar. So simple, yet so effective.

Here's my final pitch for moving to a schedule: Automating as much of your life's smaller tasks and duties frees you up to focus on bigger things. Recovering from CFS is going to require most of your attention and energy, so it's important to have everything else in your life running as smoothly as possible. By being organized and conscious about what you're doing, you'll be aware of how you are spending your time so that you can relax as much as possible and focus on the healing process.

Another thing I strongly recommend you consider implementing to reinforce the good choices you are making is to **track your progress**. This was really helpful for showing me how much and how fast my health was improving. Initially I kept it simple, using just a blank paper journal to record things, and later on I swapped that for a digital version.

Although I started by tracking things weekly, sometimes even daily, eventually I found that simply writing one paragraph every month describing what my life was like worked the best. Writing updates more often than that was time consuming and made it hard to see what progress I was making — there wasn't enough change day to day to see improvement.

It's important as well to be honest about your progress and not lie to yourself about what's happening. I would very deliberately write about what parts of my life and health were improving and what parts were still a struggle. But the best part of having a record of my progress was that, no matter where I was on my CFS recovery journey, or how slow my health gains were, I always found it inspiring to read earlier entries and see how far I'd come. Looking back and discovering specific things that at one point I couldn't do at all and could now manage easily always filled me with hope and the motivation to keep working at my healing plan.

When I first started to exercise again, I tracked the days that I did my workouts on a simple chart on my computer. It was really encouraging to see how with each passing month — regardless of how short my workouts were — I was getting in more and more days at the gym. Each month I aimed to surpass the monthly total from the last month, and this fun competition with myself helped me stay motivated and on track with my workouts.

I did something similar with my eating plan as well. If there was a particular food or drink that I was struggling to stay away from, I would commit to not having it for a certain number of weeks and tick off the successful weeks as they went by. Underneath my daily schedule in my Evernote app I'd actually put a tick box for each week I planned on abstaining. Sometimes I'd write a small message to myself underneath the numbered tick boxes to help motivate me and keep me on track. Sometimes this message was beautiful, positive, and inspiring, meant to cheer me along, like, "Today will be amazing, so wake up and smile!" Other times this message was more like a slap to the face, ordering myself to get my crap together and stop behaving like an idiot. Nothing snaps me into action like reading, "Hey, dumbass, stop wasting your one shot at a happy and healthy life." Both worked, and I seemed to know at what times I needed a cheerleading squad and when I needed a drill sergeant.

The third and final thing I'd like to recommend to move beyond the myth of willpower is to have a **checklist**. If you want to stick to your plan and ensure you are still on track, I believe the surest way to guarantee that you'll be successful is to create a checklist.

I've included one here that covers what I did to get well, but because people are all somewhat unique, you will need to customize this list and fit it to your needs. Remove the items from this list that don't speak to you. Add items that you know work well for your body. And leave room (or make it digital) so you can add things as you go — you never know what new things might come up as you move through your healing plan. You can also visit https://raelanagle.com/resources/ for a downloadable version of this checklist.

RECOVERY PLAN CHECKLIST
EXERCISE:

- I have structured my life in a way that allows regaining my health to be my number one priority.
- I have minimized my obligations so that I am free to experiment with my exercise regimen and see what works for me.
- I work out on my own so that I am not allowing pressure from myself or others to force me to do too much.
- I use the expertise found on reputable websites and mobile apps to structure my workouts.
- I follow fitness icons on social media that highlight the success stories of others to help keep me motivated and not feel alone in this journey.
- My fitness program focuses on strength training to start, and I use only my body weight or very small weights.
- I have surrendered to my limitations and, as much as possible, do not push past my limits with exercise.

- I stretch after all my workouts and again before I go to bed.
- I do what's necessary to get a good night's sleep every night

NUTRITION:

- I eat a diet filled with probiotic-rich foods such as kombucha and sauerkraut.
- I eat a predominantly whole-foods plant-based diet.
- I don't eat processed foods or foods with added sugar
- I have an organized meal-planning and food-preparation system that ensures I always have healthy meals and snacks to consume.
- If my CFS symptoms are currently severe, I don't consume any caffeine. If I have mostly recovered from CFS, I might consume some very small quantities of caffeine.
- If my CFS symptoms are currently severe, I don't consume any alcohol. If I have mostly recovered from CFS, I might occasionally consume some very small quantities of alcohol.
- I practice intermittent fasting, allowing my body to have some small breaks each day from the heavy burden of digesting and eliminating food.
- A few times per year I conduct vegetable juice cleanses lasting one–three days each.

MENTAL HEALTH:

- I do research on CFS, but I stop when I feel that what I'm reading is discouraging or unhelpful.
- I share my struggles with those close to me when needed, but I refrain from constantly complaining and repeating the same things to the people around me.
- I examine my conscious and non-conscious motives for remaining ill and ensure they are not preventing me from recovering.
- I stay away from draining people and places as much as possible.
- I am at peace with taking a step back from life while I put my focus firmly on self-care.
- I expect that both good days and bad days will be part of this recovery process and am prepared for how I will handle both.
- I meditate for at least a few minutes every day.
- I use online sources of support such as Instagram, Facebook, Twitter, and YouTube to help me cope with this process even when I'm home alone.
- I use fierce boundaries with my online content and ensure that it is positive and up lifting.
- I have found people who have achieved what I want to achieve and am learning from what worked for them.
- I spend face-to-face time with the people I care about and get the support I need.
- I laugh daily.
- I have a personalized folder of inspirational and motivational messages that I review daily.
- I cultivate gratitude for all the wonderful things I still have through the use of gratitude journals and lists.

- I use transformational vocabulary to shape my experiences in life for the better.
- I celebrate each and every success I experience along the way and document them all someplace.
- I cry when needed.
- I observe my behavior without judgement and use that information to shape my behavior for the better.
- I journal often.
- I am optimistic, but I don't let that keep me from recognizing when my plan isn't working and needs to be changed.
- I take charge of my happiness and know that the responsibility for being happy lies solely with me.

BODY SUPPORT:

- I have a consistent bedtime routine.
- I take naps when needed.
- Every day I get a healthy amount of sun.
- I take daily cold showers.
- I get regular massages.
- I listen to the messages that my body is giving me at every moment of every single day and act accordingly.

HEALING MINDSET:

- I know how to build up good habits, I am educated about what my body and mind need, and I am not in denial about any of my harmful behaviors.

- My identity is that of a strong, healthy person.
- I only place myself in environments that support my success.
- I set inspiring goals and review them regularly.
- I have an organized calendar and schedule that keep me on track every hour of every day.
- I track my progress to help me see exactly how far I've come.

Whatever you do, make a plan and stick to it. How? My suggestion is that you set a repeating reminder on your calendar to look at this checklist and make sure you are doing all the things you've committed to doing. Instead of relying on habit to get you there, a checklist reinforces that you are making conscious choices to get better. And the more you reinforce that message, over the notion that what you just need is more willpower, the better off you'll be.

19

LIFE AFTER CHRONIC FATIGUE SYNDROME

Finally overcoming CFS feels nothing short of miraculous, and regaining my health is by far the biggest accomplishment of my life. Life with this disease compared to a life without it is like comparing night and day. The chains that for so many years kept holding me back and keeping me down are finally gone. My ten-year flu has finally ended, and at last, I feel completely free to live my life in the manner in which it was always meant to be lived.

Yet while struggling with chronic fatigue syndrome, as much as I desperately wanted to get past it, there was a part of me that surprisingly felt a little reluctant to leave the struggle behind. This was a decade-long battle, and for all those years, whether I liked it or not, this illness was so much a part of who I was. Getting past CFS and then simply moving on with life as if none of it ever happened felt a bit like working my butt off to get an invisible PhD. I would have nothing to show for all these years of struggle other than being *normal*.

As much as I wanted to move past this illness, I knew something about it wasn't sitting well with me. I wasn't sure how I was supposed to just go on and live the rest of my life as if none of this had ever happened. I wasn't sure how to finally put CFS down and walk away from it for good.

I realize now that just because you get past the struggle, it doesn't mean that it never happened. Once you get past it, the strength, knowledge, and resilience you gained in the process stay with you and shine through in everything you do for the rest of your life. The good parts of it stay parts of you, making you a better person and more equipped in everything you do. I feel tougher. I am a fighter. I know what I want. I know who I am.

So what now?

Let's start with the bad.

Although I've come out the other side of CFS in a much better place than I was before this all started, there are definitely some residual struggles that I still face. For one, now that I'm past this illness I seem to think I should be past all forms of illness for good. Since I've put in my time with suffering and I've worked so hard to get healthy, I seem to think that I am impervious to being sick, and as a result, I am blindsided whenever any small bouts of illness come my way. Although you'd think that my past marathon of illness would have resulted in some sort of endurance in this area, now that I'm past CFS my patience and tolerance for suffering are actually almost nonexistent.

How this hurts me is that, when the odd cold or flu inevitably comes my way, I have trouble slowing down. Not wanting to spend another day of my life laid out on the couch, I keep pushing through my daily activities, and as a result, it takes me much longer to get better than it should. It doesn't even occur to me that, for both my sake and others, I should cancel any plans I have. During my years with CFS, if I canceled my plans every time I didn't feel well, I never would have gone anywhere, with anyone, ever. I have over a decade's worth of experience with powering through things, and this has proven to be an incredibly challenging habit to put down.

Yet whereas I'm proud of myself for showing up to the girl's weekend brunch despite my sniffles and nagging cough, the people around me are less thrilled to be exposed to my walking petri dish of communicable illness. And because I'm not at home resting like I should be, my poor body has a big job to do in trying to overcome whatever it's battling.

I also struggle to admit and accept that this world of over-achieving entrepreneurs isn't for me. There's so much out there, from books and online sources, that drive home the importance of squeezing out as many productive hours each week as possible and getting in those eighteen-hour days. I am wired for efficiency, and accepting that, for me, efficiency involves sufficient downtime and relaxation is a tough one.

As much as my mind might be wired to do all of that, I just can't risk the devastating health implications for my body that can come with that kind of lifestyle. My hard-earned freedom comes hand-in-hand with a vigilance for self-care on which I don't think I will ever ease up. And as alluring as it might be to be that person who publishes countless books, has non-stop high-quality YouTube videos, travels the world to attend and speak at conferences, and has her own clothing line, I just don't think that that can ever be me.

I love the infectious enthusiasm put out by so many go-get-'em influencers out there telling us to work out twice per day and never stop trying to squeeze more productive hours out of our days, but I just can't be a part of all that. As great as I feel, I remain a little bit scared of life and what it can do to me. Crappy, but true. I suspect that ten years of illness would make even the strongest and most resilient of folks a tad gun shy. I imagine that as my healthy years accumulate these feelings of fear will ease up, but until then I need to find my own way and develop my own recipe for living life to the fullest and never stop believing that I can have an exceptional life in spite of my slightly dialed-back efforts. Despite now feeling completely energetic and healthy, I've seen what can happen when I push myself too hard, and I don't ever want to risk having to experience that kind of illness and suffering ever again. Been there. Done that. Lesson learned.

Now, let's talk about the good!

It's an amazing and beautiful thing how quickly I was able to put the bulk of the pain down, to move on with my life, and to leave the trauma behind me. As challenging as it was at times, life with CFS shaped and molded me into the person I am proud to be today. Even though I might still hold back a bit, I came out of this whole experience acutely aware of the joy of fully living. I now seize every opportunity for happiness, adventure, friendship, and love.

Overcoming CFS isn't a one-time transformation. Nothing stops just because I'm better. The dedicated regimen of self-care I developed to combat CFS is my new normal. Prioritizing my health, both physical and mental, is something on which I am no longer willing to compromise. I might be flexible in my methods, but I remain firm in making myself a priority. Once you see what life feels like living in a healthy and strong body that you can rely on and be proud of every second of every day, there is absolutely no going back.

The good news about CFS and any residual fear that might remain after healing is that it forces you to live the best version of your life possible. Keeping up all of that self-care is now both easy and fun. Before CFS, I tried so hard to eat well and get in shape, but I just couldn't quite figure out how to put it all together successfully. Food is just easy for me now and so incredibly enjoyable! There is no stress around deciding what to eat or what not to eat. I am no longer at war with food and am free to simply appreciate it as the beautiful instrument of nourishment that it is.

The same is true about exercise. I *love* to exercise. I am straight-up pumped up with excitement every single day when I open up my exercise app and get to see what my workout is for that day. (I actually have to keep myself from opening the app the night before and peaking because I want to save the excitement of the big reveal for the morning of my workout.) The feeling of my active body showing me how capable and strong it is is a drug. Exercise no longer leaves me feeling drained or causes suffering in any way. It leaves me feeling strong, confident, and equipped to take on anything.

And all those skills I learned for managing stress, developing good habits, and finding joy are just as useful today as they ever were. Life, as life does, still occasionally throws crap at me, but having the mental toughness to deal with it all just makes everything go so much more smoothly. I use all of those skills I cultivated to help me succeed in every area of my life. Once you've developed the ability to manage your life with CFS, then taking on this world without it becomes a walk in the park.

When this is all said and done, you will look and feel the best you ever have.

I wish I could say with absolute certainty that CFS is behind me forever, but the truth is I can't. Although I've figured out how to heal from CFS, I still don't fully understand the mechanisms of how it works. Is it still lingering in my body somewhere, hiding in the shadows and waiting to make a comeback? Unfortunately, I really can't say for sure. What I do believe, with every ounce of my being, is that if it is lurking someplace in my body, by continuing to do the things that got me well I will also be able to continue to keep it at bay. I would never take a chance and trash my body again like I used to in the past, because I don't ever want to allow my health to fall into disrepair ever again.

And just because CFS is no longer an issue, that doesn't mean that my body isn't still faced with other stressors. With so much toxicity in this world, it's a full-time job for our bodies to keep themselves clean, strong, and healthy. All the practices I learned for supporting my body, such as fasting, eating fermented foods, enjoying a primarily whole-foods plant-based diet, getting some sun, taking cold showers, and getting massages, still serve my body today. I want to make sure that my body continues to thrive and stays in this blissful state of vibrant health for the rest of my life.

I hate chronic fatigue syndrome. Truly and deeply I do. It is a devastating life-demolisher that I wouldn't wish on anyone. It is debilitating, and it is destructive. It is every kind of bad.

But. There is no denying that CFS brought me an extraordinary life and made me a significantly better person than I was before I got it. Even in the midst of the worst parts of my suffering, I could see that I was going to come out the other end of this a much better person because I got sick.

While preparing to write this book, I went back and read my journals from my first couple years with CFS, and one entry that stood out to me was written during my first year of being sick. At this point I'd already been off work for eight months, and despite how many different things in my life (job, gym, social life) had come to a screeching halt, I wrote that I had not yet felt bored for even one second. Despite often being housebound and mostly alone, for months I'd managed to keep myself feeling engaged and entertained every single day.

During that time, I read so incredibly much. I learned so much. I journaled and journaled and then journaled some more. CFS served as a personal growth bootcamp in which I was learning in months what otherwise would have taken me years. Most of us think we can take a two-week vacation to recharge and get some perspective on the direction we want our lives to take. At that point in my life, two weeks wouldn't even have scratched the surface.

CFS for me was a heavily disguised life coach. During every day that I was paying attention, there was a lesson for me to learn. I see now that before I got sick, so much of the life that I was living didn't match who I actually was. During that screeching halt of CFS, I got to see through and get past the internal and external pressures that pushed me to try to be something that I wasn't. This sickness turned out to be a strange and unusual gift that launched me into the life I truly wanted to be living.

When I read through my journals from my years of being sick, I want to scream with excitement through the pages at that poor sick girl about all the unbelievable things that are to come. Wow, the adventures that await! Unbelievable joy and bliss are waiting. So so much was, and still is, to come.

I would never want (or expect anyone else) to be thankful for suffering. But I do think that it's important to take these moments of struggle and get the most you can from them. They have a way of catapulting our personal growth in ways that are quite challenging to achieve when things are going smoothly.

As nasty as it can be, CFS can also be a bearer of incredible gifts. This illness, and how I chose to deal with it, brought me my dream life. It got me to sit still long enough to examine how I was living and find the courage to make drastic changes and fix the things that needed fixing. It showed me that everything can be taken away in an instant, so there is no point in living a life that isn't truly what you want.

Would I have achieved some of these things without CFS? Probably. But I know the path I was on before CFS hit, and I can pretty much guarantee that I wouldn't have achieved most of them. Before illness turned my world upside down I didn't at all have the focus, the clarity, or the courage I needed to pursue my dreams.

CFS pushed me to find a way to travel the world for years and to live in so many different countries. I've met amazing people from all over the globe and developed so many cherished friendships. I followed my passion for art and learned how to paint. I fulfilled a lifelong dream of learning how to surf. I discovered a new passion that I didn't even know I had when I became a professional scuba diver. I got to experience the exhausting yet exhilarating process of becoming a writer, and in connecting with others who are

their health I found one of my true passions
n life.

rned how to relax, how to minimize stress, and
really important in life. I learned how to say no, to
to myself. I learned about the importance of quieting
my mind and about stepping back and powering down once in
a while. I learned about the value of connecting with nature. I
learned how to put my mind in tune with my body, allowing
me to hear the messages my body sends about what it needs to
thrive. I learned how to be my own health advocate and not
accept information from anyone that I intuitively know to be
false for me. I learned to take care of myself, whether anyone
else thinks it's necessary or not.

I learned how to cherish and be present for the people I
care about in my life and to not worry so much about what the
rest think. I learned about drawing boundaries and enforcing
them and about setting limits for myself and others. I learned
about the importance of daily joy and laughter and about the
devastating impacts of stress. I learned about my limitations,
that they exist and that I need to accept that I have them. I
learned that it's ok at times to be weak, to not be able to do it all,
and to have others be aware of that.

I developed a healthy relationship with food and finally
understand how it really does fuel us and determine our quality
of life. I learned to face my addictions and that they do not, in
fact, control me.

I learned about the incredibly awesome power of
reframing things in life. I realized that many things that I
thought were so incredibly important weren't that important
at all. I learned that my value is in no way determined by the
size of my house and that maybe, just maybe, my true beauty
is on the inside. I learned that I am a valuable, worthy individual who should at all times hold my head up high. I learned

that I can learn something from every person that I meet. I learned how to face my fears and that most aren't nearly as terrifying as I once thought they were. I learned about the importance of living in the moment, because that's all I ever really have.

When I first got sick with CFS, it was like driving a trusted car that suddenly broke down on the side of the road, leaving me stranded and needing to walk for miles in order to get back home. So for a while, I stopped trusting that car, because that car no longer felt safe or like something that I could rely on. But instead of giving up on driving completely, I learned as much as I could about what could possibly be wrong and then went back to that car and worked on it until I figured out how to fix it.

Moving forward, despite my cautious attitude toward self-care, I won't live in fear of another CFS engine failure, because now I have the knowledge, experience, and skills to tackle whatever problems come up next. As a result of that breakdown, I've learned how to be my own mechanic. I've gained a much greater understanding of my body, and that feeling of having no control over what happens to my health has largely disappeared. Now I listen to my body, I pay attention to the warning lights, and I take care of things before they get to a state of emergency. I treat my body with the care and respect for which it's been begging for ages, and now that I've got its back, it always has mine too.

With the prison of CFS behind me, I cherish and embrace every single moment of my freedom. The possibilities for me, for my life, are now endless.

If CFS is still holding back you or someone you care about, let me know how I can help. Email me, find me on Instagram, or touch base on Facebook. Reach out on Twitter or find me on YouTube. Just somehow, somewhere, take action and get in touch, because I would be honored to be there for you and be a part of your healing story. There are so many of us out there needlessly suffering alone, and it's time that we join hands and beat this together.

CONCLUSION
YOU'VE GOT THIS!

I know that life with CFS can be really draining and daunting, and it can feel at times like you will never be free of it. What's worse is that life with CFS can start to feel normal. After I'd been living with CFS for a while, I came to a place where for a long time I just stopped fighting. Life with CFS was my new normal. But it's important to remember that a normal, healthy life actually looks nothing like a life with chronic illness. That a life with chronic fatigue syndrome is absolutely unacceptable. You get what you tolerate, and you need to decide that you will not tolerate CFS in your life any longer.

People do fully recover from chronic fatigue syndrome. Know this. Internalize this. Carve these words into your soul as the absolute truth. If you currently suffer from CFS, you need to decide right now that you don't want to suffer anymore. That you want to fully live and enjoy your life. That each day can no longer be a burden to bear.

Aside from CFS, the biggest enemy you'll face in this will be yourself. The minute you start to doubt that your efforts are actually taking you where you want to go is the minute that things will fall apart. Life might throw in some obstacles along the way, but if your belief in yourself and in the process is unshakable, then absolutely nothing will keep you from getting you to where you want to go.

In the beginning, I had to rely on optimism and positive thinking to keep me going, but once I could see that what I was doing was working, that I was actually getting better, optimism wasn't a part of the equation anymore. I didn't have to hope I would get better — an honest and objective assessment of the facts served up my unshakable motivation to keep going.

It's normal to worry that you might fail and to feel anxiety about putting in this monstrous amount of effort. It's normal to have doubts — to ask yourself *what if it doesn't work?* But the real question you should be asking yourself is *what if it does?* Can you really, truly imagine what your life could be like? I bet you can. Imagine the possibilities! Imagine what life will feel like with no limits. When each day is an inspiring new endeavor to be enjoyed.

It's not always easy; that's for sure. Nothing worth having ever is, and this is no different. Hard work and determination are essential. Keep your eye on the prize and keep plugging along. No matter how difficult your life with CFS might be, you can't let despair win. You have to fight for the life you deserve. You have to listen to that internal voice telling you what you need and keep doing that until you are truly free.

But you have to choose to be free. Hope is not a strategy. What are you going to do today that will ensure you are a little closer to reaching your goals by bedtime? What are you going to do to ensure that every single morning you can celebrate the fact that in some small but significant way you are stronger than yesterday? Whatever you do, always put in your best, and recognize your best will vary. And that forward is forward, no matter how slow.

It took me years before I once again finally made the choice to go all-in and work to get better. It wasn't too late for me, and it's not too late for you. Nor is it the wrong time. You're not too old/young/sick/broke/busy/depressed to get started. Where ever you are right now, in this exact moment as you are reading these words, is the absolute best time to get started. If you've made it this far in my book, then you're definitely ready to choose your health. As they say, *If the best time to plant a tree was twenty years ago, the second-best time is now.*

Many of us live in places where junk food-filled sedentary lives are the norm. Where not taking care of ourselves is the norm. This is not the path to your best life. It's time to admit some hard truths when it comes to what's holding you back. To admit that we ourselves are what's holding us back. Now is the time to stop lying to yourself, thinking you're some special exception that can trash your body and not follow a healing plan and somehow still miraculously feel great.

Just imagine where you could be this time next year if you decided to start today. The time is going to pass no matter what, so you might as well do something great with it! It's up to you where you'll find yourself a year from now.

Just start by tackling some manageable chunks, and in time, what is manageable will increase. My daily schedule, now fairly packed full of activities, used to mostly be blocked off for rest. I would sleep and lie on the couch with my greasy hair and the clothes I slept in and just read or watch Netflix. To get to where I am now I started out really small. First I added one minute of exercise per day, along with occasionally going to the grocery store across the street to buy some kombucha, sauerkraut, and some healthy pre-made meals. In time, I was able to actually start making my own kombucha and some basic homemade healthy dinners and still feel ok. Then I found I had enough energy to make the sauerkraut myself too, on top of working out five minutes per day. Then ten. Then fifteen. Before long I was even showering on a regular basis and occasionally even wearing normal clothes. With each and every passing week, by listening to my body and taking care of it in the ways that are proven to be successful and made sense to me, I got closer and closer to where I wanted to be.

Once you get started, I know it can be really easy to get off track. Sometimes we find a recipe for success, try it, find out it works, and then slowly start to abandon the recipe, thinking that success will somehow remain without us putting in any more effort. Health is never owned, it is rented, and the rent is due every day. Don't lose focus. Keep your eye on the prize. You're on a great path right now. Stay on it! It'll take you amazing places. You need to stick this out because it is *so* worth the effort.

Getting past CFS can feel a bit like running a marathon. In any long race, there is a stretch in the middle where motivation and belief in yourself might start to wane. It's relatively easy to be pumped when the race kicks off, while the excitement is still fresh and your adrenaline is pumping strong. And I doubt that many runners give up once that finish line is concretely in their line of sight. It's in that long, winding, draining section in the middle where I picture that motivation and belief in yourself might start to dwindle.

When battling an opponent like CFS, it can be tempting to quit before you're done. Once you've been working on your healing plan for a while and seen some significant progress with your health, it might be tempting to take a step back from your healing regimen for a bit. You might have more energy and the demands of life might be calling, and even though you are not yet 100 percent recovered from CFS, you think that you can't possibly justify spending any more time focusing just on yourself. You might think, *I've made enough progress for the time being; let's just see how I do going back to work.*

I've quit my healing plan before I was done a few times along the way, so I know firsthand some of the ways this can go. The worst that will happen is that you'll act like you're fully recovered and then crater like a meteorite has hit you. I've definitely been there and done that! I naively jumped back into a full-time job *way* before I was ready, and as a result, I crashed hard and undid all the progress I'd made with my health. After a few months of this, I had to quit my job and then had to spend six months in bed simply recovering from what I did. Not six months where I was getting better — six months of putting on the breaks to stop my downward slide so I could turn the train around and get pointed in the right direction once again. I'd put myself into a devastating physical and emotional slump that was incredibly difficult to pull myself out of.

The best-case scenario is that your health stays exactly where it is. (I think you know by now that it's not going to keep on miraculously improving on its own.) If you are 50, 60, maybe 70 percent better, then that's where you will stay. This happened to me once. I didn't get worse, but I didn't get one iota better either. And although I appeared to be a relatively healthy and functional person on the surface, I struggled to keep up with *everything* in my life, and most days I was hanging on by a thread.

I often read about people with CFS who recover about 70 percent but who never seem to be able to get any further than that, and I suspect something similar is happening with them. It's understandable that once you've seen some progress you'd be tempted to take on some of your old responsibilities or add some new ones. Guilt kicks in, and the demands of life start screaming at you more loudly, and the bills are piling up. So you change your focus from internal to external, and before you know it your healing plan has taken a back seat to everything else.

But I'm telling you that even if you've recovered 70 percent of your health, there is still *so much* missing. Recovering that last 30 percent is a total game-changer. As tempting as I know it can be, don't quit before you're at the finish line. That portion of your health that is still missing is significant, and every day it will hold you back and make far too much of your life feel like a burden to endure. A cage that is 70 percent larger than it was before is still a cage.

So keep going. If you quit on yourself you will *never* get past the things that you are struggling with. When you're almost there, that last bit will be the part that completely transforms your life.

At times it felt like my whole life revolved around my trying to get better, and some days I just felt so cut off from the world. With all the rest and recovery time needed, healing from CFS was sometimes a lonely process. Without the activity and excitement of having a job, an active social life, and all the other daily distractions that come with a healthy life, sometimes the loneliness and isolation could be suffocating.

When I felt like I might just lose my mind if I didn't go do something, then regardless of my energy levels, I'd go do something. Sometimes we just really need a break. And these breaks, despite how much they might've drained my energy reserves, did wonders for replenishing my reserves of happiness and my motivation to keep going.

It's ok to take breaks once in a while during this fight, but don't ever quit completely. It's ok to not be relentlessly positive all the time, but don't give up. Just don't give up and don't quit. The incredible payoff for all your efforts is just around the corner. And in times of doubt, listen for your internal voice of infinite wisdom that knows the truth of what you need to do.

In Robert Kiyosaki's book *Rich Dad Poor Dad,* he explains that even if people have all the financial information they need, there are things that can prevent them from getting on top of their finances. Unfortunately, sometimes even when we know how to do something, cynicism and even arrogance can keep us from being successful.

I believe that this is true when it comes to getting on top of our health as well. Toward the end of my mother's journey with CFS, she had mostly given up on the idea of ever getting well. If I found new information on treating CFS or suggested new things to try, she would usually quickly shoot these ideas down. I suspect that after decades of trying different things without success, she was scared to get her hopes up again. She was probably skeptical that anything would work and had become pretty cynical about her health in general. She'd also developed a whole host of bad habits such as smoking and eating unhealthy foods that she seemed reluctant to give up. It's an understandable state of mind to be in, but not a helpful one.

My worst habit is a slight tendency toward arrogance. I sometimes think I can do this alone, and then I start making promises to myself I wind up not keeping. I found my battle with CFS to be a great time to develop some personal integrity. I learned to not break promises to myself and to be the number one person in my life I could rely on to get things done. When I said I was going to do something, I did it. This had always been true when it came to promises I'd make to other people, but now it was true for myself as well.

The issue with silent, undocumented promises to ourselves is that if we break them, we can easily pretend that we never even made these promises in the first place. To help break this habit of letting myself down, I learned to start saying the promises I'd made to myself out loud to other people. This got my ego involved, and since I didn't want to look like a fool, by telling someone else my plans it became pretty certain that I'd follow through. I'd also write my promise to myself down some-place that I would see it every day. By writing it down and saying it out loud, I couldn't pretend the promise didn't exist.

If you've done a ton of research and know how to shape your habits and environment to make yourself successful, but still aren't achieving your goals, it might be worth taking a look to see if you've become cynical or arrogant.

You're almost at the end of this book, and you know what you have to do. You don't want to choose a life of suffering. It might be hard, and you might not see results instantly. But they are coming, and you have to keep pushing like the completely unstoppable force that you know you are. You have so much to gain — and so much to lose if you do nothing. A life of suffering does not have to be your destiny. Not if you don't let it.

As one of my biggest role models in life Rachel Hollis insists, you are not defined by the pain life inflicts — you are defined by what you turn that pain into. Will you allow it to make you bitter? Skeptical? Jaded? Will you allow it to erode your joy? Will you allow CFS to keep you from living your full life? Rachel and I both hope not.[1]

Just start where you are, use what you have, and do what you can. Stop being your own greatest critic and start being your own greatest fan. Focus on what you *can* do instead of what you can't. Each day that you're taking care of yourself and doing all these beautiful things to help your body recover is a day that you're making progress. And trust that the progress is happening, even if you can't immediately see it. Whatever you do, just get to work.

And know that although I've shared the recipe detailing what worked for me to find my freedom again, everyone's experience with recovery is deeply individual, as is their decision on how to heal. Take from my story what makes sense to you and leave the rest, because in and of itself, learning to recognize the things that aren't meant for you is a vital part of your way out of this.

Like it has for me, this journey can connect you to other amazing like-minded people, people whose stories will inspire you and motivate you to stay on the path that you need to be on. This struggle connects us on some level that I can't hope to ever understand or explain. But you know it and you feel it.

If you've been alone in this fight until now, rest assured that you've found that connection you seek. When life feels impossible you'll feel this tribe, our tribe of warriors, there with you every step of the way to lift you up. Feel us in your heart. Visit https://raelanagle.com , or say hello on Instagram @raelan.agle, or check out my weekly YouTube videos (on my channel creatively named Raelan Agle) to keep learning more about the topics covered in this book and connect with other amazing individuals who have conquered CFS all over the world.

Your story has power. Share it. The world needs your energy. You never know who is paying attention and waiting for a little inspiration. And whatever you do, never forget that we are here for you, we are here *with* you, and we know that you've got this.

PHOTOGRAPHS

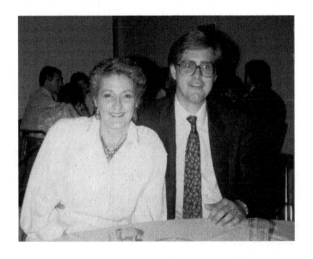

My parents Patricia Agle and Brian Agle.

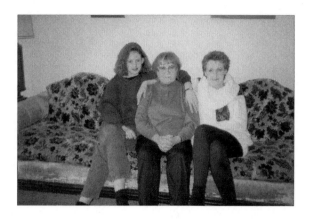

Left to right: Myself, my maternal grandmother Jean Fedechko, and my mother Patricia Agle.

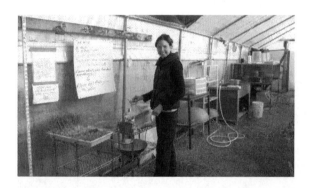

Me making wheatgrass juice at the rejuvenation center in the desert.

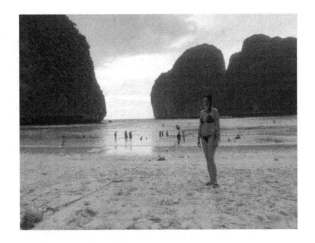

Me at "The Beach" in Koh Phi Phi Le, Thailand.

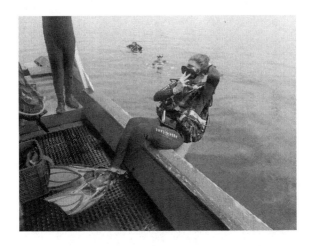

Me as a professional scuba diver in Southeast Asia.

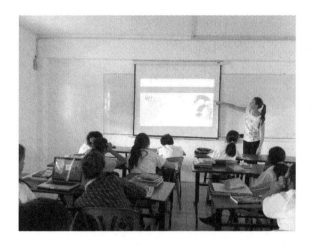

Me teaching in Kuala Lumpur, Malaysia.

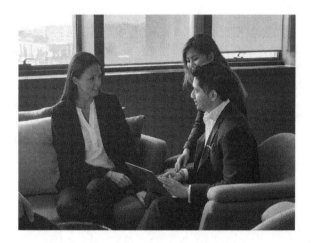

Me at my corporate job in Kuala Lumpur, Malaysia.

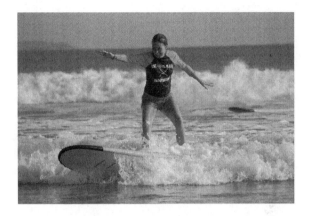

Me learning to surf in Bali, Indonesia.

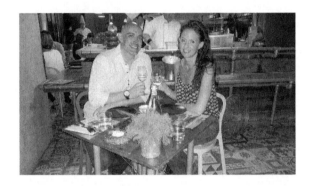

My first date with Geoffrey in Kuala Lumpur, Malaysia.

Thanks so much for reading! Truly. If you loved the book and have a moment to spare, a nice way to say thanks is to write a short online review, as this helps out indie authors such as myself immensely and helps new readers to find my book!

Still want to learn more? Visit raelanagle.com to sign up for my email list and discover more tools for living your happiest and healthiest life.

APPENDIX A

APPENDIX A

SUGGESTED APPS

SWEAT: a fitness app available on your mobile phone where some prominent fitness trainers have programs available for use at home or at a gym. At the time of writing this, the cost is one hundred and twenty US dollars for a yearly subscription and twenty dollars per month for a monthly subscription.

CENTR: a personalized health and fitness app. At the time of writing this, the cost is one hundred and twenty US dollars for a yearly subscription and twenty dollars per month for a monthly subscription.

ANYLIST: a mobile app great for making organized grocery lists. Free at the time of this writing.

HEADSPACE: a meditation and mindfulness mobile app with both free and various paid options.

EVERNOTE: a note-taking mobile and desktop app great for organizing lists and schedules with both free and paid options.

PINTEREST: a mobile and desktop social media app great for finding recipes. Free at the time of this writing.

ACKNOWLEDGMENTS

I am fortunate that there are quite a few people who helped bring this book to life. Foremost, I am grateful to my wonderful partner in life, Geoffrey Hussey, for being my rock while I took the time off work to both finally recover from CFS and then also write a book about it. I suspect he spent as many hours listening to me talk about this book as I spent writing it, and for his unremitting support and patience with this and all the other awesomeness he possesses I will be forever grateful.

Thank you to my editor Dr. D. Olson Pook (https://dolsonpook.com) whose brilliant insights and suggestions guided me in how to best tell my story and help others in the process. For his patience and the skilled manner in which he handled this first-time writer I will forever be grateful. Thank you also to Megan Nicole Swenson for doing the proofreading and providing some additional tweaks to help make this book the best that it could be. Thank you to Miladinka Milic (www.milagraphicartist.com) for designing the cover. I am thankful also to my friend Mohamed Elbadwihi who early on generously donated his time and creative talents to help me explore the design elements of this book. A huge thank you to my dear friend Natalia Howat who has been my ceaseless supporter and this book's number-one fan from the time when it was barely a few poorly strung together words on my laptop and right up until the very end. Much gratitude also to my beta readers Natalia Howat, Panida Grinneback, Jennifer Kardynal, Janice Anderson, Jasmine Champion, Samantha Etchells, Alexandra Fedechko, Melanie Tay, Jennifer Moran, Jody-Lynn Twele, Stella Tran, and Devona Crnkovic for volunteering their time to read and provide vital feedback on my story before I released it to the world.

Without the ongoing support of my father, Brian Agle, I would not be where I am today. He always has my back and consistently makes me feel loved and that I am never alone in this world. I don't know how I can ever possibly hope to repay him for all that he's done and continues to do in the manner in which he deserves.

I'm also sending love and gratitude to my mother, who I held close to my heart while I wrote every page of this book. Even though she's gone, I know how ecstatic and how proud she would be that I'm sharing our stories with the hopes of helping others.

And finally, a humongous thank you to you, the reader, because most of all I was always writing this for you.

ABOUT THE AUTHOR

ABOUT THE AUTHOR

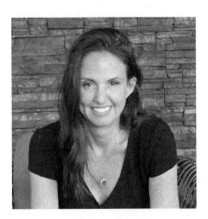

Raelan Agle has a Master's degree in social work from Dalhousie University and worked as a social worker in her home country of Canada before leaving to embrace her passion for exploring the world. She has since visited dozens of countries and lived in six, including her current home in San Francisco, USA. Despite her lack of formal medical training, when doctors couldn't help her recover from a debilitating chronic illness she did her own research and found a way to cure herself. She now has an emerging following as a lifestyle influencer on social media where she works to share her hard-earned lessons on health, healing, and happiness for the benefit of others. Visit raelanagle.com to find out about her latest projects and passions.

REFERENCE LIST

"About · Deliciously Ella." *Deliciously Ella*, https:// deliciouslyella.com/about/.

Campbell-McBride, Natasha. *Gut and Psychology Syndrome*. Medinform Publishing, 2012.

"Can Caffcine Relieve Your Chronic Fatigue?" *Everyday-Health.com*, 4 Mar. 2010, https://www.everydayhealth.com/ chronic-fatigue-syndrome/relief-with-caffeine.aspx.

Clear, James. *Atomic Habits: An Easy & Proven Way to Build Good Habits & Break Bad Ones*. Avery Publishing Group, 2018.

Crowley, Chris, and Henry S. Lodge. *Younger next Year: a Guide to Living like 50 until You're 80 and Beyond*. Workman Pub., 2007.

"Don't Get Sabotaged by Added Sugar." *Mayo Clinic*, Mayo Foundation for Medical Education and Research, 30 Jan. 2019, https://www.mayoclinic.org/healthy-lifestyle/nutrition-and-healthy-eating/in-depth/added-sugar/art-20045328.

"Eating You Alive™." *Eating You Alive™*, https://www. eatingyoualive.com/.

Edward R. Laskowski, M.D. "Are Isometric Exercises Good for Strength Training?" *Mayo Clinic*, Mayo Foundation for Medical Education and Research, 17 Jan. 2018, https://www.mayoclinic.org/healthy-lifestyle/fitness/expert-answers/isometric-exercises/faq-20058186.

"Effects of Alcohol on the Body and the Brain." *Alcohol Rehab Guide*, https://www.alcoholrehabguide.org/alcohol/effects/.

"Fasting." *Wikipedia*, Wikimedia Foundation, 7 Oct. 2019, https://en.wikipedia.org/wiki/Fasting.

Films, A.U.M. "WHAT THE HEALTH." *WHAT THE HEALTH*, http://www.whatthehealthfilm.com/.

Flynn, Patrick. *I Disagree: How These Two Words Are the Secret to Thinking Differently and Taking Control of Your Health*.

"Get Enough Sleep." *Healthfinder.gov*, https://health.gov/myhealthfinder/topics/everyday-healthy-living/mental-health-and-relationships/get-enough-sleep

Grace, Annie. *This Naked Mind: Control Alcohol, Find Freedom, Discover Happiness & Change Your Life*. Avery, an Imprint of Penguin Random House, 2018.

HARDY, BENJAMIN. *WILLPOWER DOESNT WORK: Discover the Hidden Keys to Success*. HACHETTE Books, 2019.

Harvard Health Publishing. "Benefits of Moderate Sun Exposure." *Harvard Health*, https://www.health.harvard.edu/diseases-and-conditions/benefits-of-moderate-sun-exposure.

Hollis, Rachel. *Didn't See That Coming: Putting Life back Together When Your World Falls Apart*. Hey St., An Imprint of William Morrow, 2020.

Hughes, Locke. "How Does Too Much Sugar Affect Your Body?" *WebMD*, WebMD, https://www.webmd.com/diabetes/features/how-sugar-affects-your-body.

Ilgunas, Ken. *Walden on Wheels: on the Open Road from Debt to Freedom*. New Harvest, Houghton Mifflin Harcourt, 2013.

"Juicer Buying Guide." *FOOD MATTERS®*, https://www.foodmatters.com/juicer-buying-guide.

Kiyosaki, Robert T., and Sharon L. Lechter. *Rich Dad, Poor Dad. What the Rich Teach Their Kids about Money-That the Poor and Middle Class Do Not!* Warner, 2000.

"List of Suicide Crisis Lines." *Wikipedia*, Wikimedia Foundation, 10 Sept. 2019, https://en.wikipedia.org/wiki/List_of_suicide_crisis_lines.

"Lymphatic System: Facts, Functions & Diseases." *LiveScience*, Purch, https://www.livescience.com/26983-lymphatic-system.html.

Margery, and Margery. "He Who Blames Others Has A Long Way To Go On His Journey." *The Minds Journal*, 5 Apr. 2018, https://themindsjournal.com/blames-others-long-way-go-journey/.

"Mel's Former Account (@Melrobbinslive) • Instagram Photos and Videos." *Instagram*, https://www.instagram.com/melrobbinslive/.

"Netflix." *KonMari*, https://konmari.com/pages/netflix.

"Overviews of Diseases/Conditions | Overviews of Diseases/Conditions | Tips From Former Smokers | CDC." *Centers for Disease Control and Prevention*, Centers for Disease Control and Prevention, https://www.cdc.gov/tobacco/campaign/tips/diseases/index.html

Repinski, Karyn. "The Health Benefits of Some Sun Exposure." *Consumer Reports*, https://www.consumerreports.org/health-wellness/sun-exposure-health-benefits/.

Robbins, Anthony. *Awaken the Giant Within: How to Take Immediate Control of Your Mental, Emotional, Physical & Financial Destiny*. Simon & Schuster Paperbacks, 2013.

"Sabbatical." *Dictionary.com*, Dictionary.com, https://www.dictionary.com/browse/sabbatical.

"Saving Your Own Life." *Psychology Today*, Sussex Publishers, https://www.psychologytoday.com/intl/blog/the-chronicles-infertility/201809/saving-your-own-life.

"Sleep Deprivation and Deficiency." *National Heart Lung and Blood Institute*, US Department of Health and Human Services, https://www.nhlbi.nih.gov/health-topics/sleep-deprivation-and-deficiency.

Spector, Tim. *Diet Myth – the Real Science behind What We Eat*. Orion Publishing Co, 2016.

Spence, David., Jenkins, David., & Davignon, Jean. Egg Yolk Consumption and Carotid Plaque. *Atherosclerosis Journal*, Oct. 2012, https://www.atherosclerosis-journal.com/article/S0021-9150(12)00504-7/abstract

Taubes, Gary. "Is Sugar Toxic?" *The New York Times*, The New York Times, 13 Apr. 2011, https://www.nytimes.com/2011/04/17/magazine/mag-17Sugar-t.html.

Watson, Stephanie. "Cross Training: Benefits, Intensity Level, and More." *WebMD*, WebMD, https://www.webmd.com/fitness-exercise/a-z/cross-training.

"What Is Calisthenics?: The School of Calisthenics Explains." *School of Calisthenics*, https://schoolofcalisthenics.com/learn-calisthenics/what-is-calisthenics/.

Why I Quit Paleo Ketogenic Diet & Went Plant-Based – Dr. Lim.https://www.youtube.com/watch?v=tbH6TIdtZ3Q.

Woolley, James, et al. "Alcohol Use in Chronic Fatigue Syndrome." *Journal of Psychosomatic Research*, U.S. National Library of Medicine, Feb. 2004, https://www.ncbi.nlm.nih.gov/pubmed/15016579.

NOTES

Preface

1. Rachel Hollis, "Didn't See That Coming"

7. Gathering Your Healing Fuel

1. *Eating You Alive* was another documentary that elaborated on and supported everything that the doctors were saying about a WFPB diet in *What the Health*.
2. Spence, Jenkins, & Davignon Egg yolk consumption and carotid plaque

8. Taking A Break

1. Food Matters, "Juicer Buying Guide"

9. The Fantastically Bad Four

1. CDC, "Overviews of Diseases/Conditions"
2. Hughes, "How Does Too Much Sugar Affect Your Body"
3. Taubes, "Is Sugar Toxic?"
4. Mayo Clinic, "Added Sugars: Don't get sabotaged by sweeteners"
5. Galbicsek, "Effects of Alcohol"
6. Myers, "Can Caffeine Relieve Your Chronic Fatigue?"

10. Making Food Work For You

1. Woolley, Allen, & Wesseley, "Alcohol Use in Chronic Fatigue Syndrome"

12. Carrying Out Your Exercise Program

1. School of Calisthenics, "What is Calisthenics"
2. Watson, "Cross Training"
3. Laskowski, "Are isometric exercises a good way to build strength?"

13. Becoming Your Body's Ally

1. National Heart, Lung, and Blood Institute, "Sleep Deprivation and Deficiency"
2. National Heart, Lung, and Blood Institute, "Sleep Deprivation and Deficiency"
3. U.S. Department of Health and Human Services, "Get Enough Sleep"
4. Repinski, "The Health Benefits of Some Sun Exposure"
5. Harvard Health Publishing, "Benefits of Moderate Sun Exposure"
6. Repinski, "The Health Benefits of Some Sun Exposure"
7. Zimmermann, "Lymphatic System: Facts, Functions, and Diseases"

15. Balancing Your Emotions

1. Ornish & Ornish, "Undo it! How Simple Lifestyle Changes Can Reverse the Onset of Most Chronic Diseases"
2. Ornish & Ornish, "Undo it! How Simple Lifestyle Changes Can Reverse the Onset of Most Chronic Diseases"

16. Habits For Happiness

1. Ornish & Ornish, "Undo it! How Simple Lifestyle Changes Can Reverse the Onset of Most Chronic Diseases"

17. The Myth Of Willpower

1. James Clear, Atomic Habits: An Easy & Proven Way to Build Good Habits & Break Bad Ones

Conclusion

1. Rachel Hollis, "Didn't See That Coming"

Manufactured by Amazon.ca
Bolton, ON

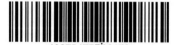

40375477R00179